Needle Core Biopsy of Lymph Nodes

Needle Core Biopsy of Lymph Nodes

An Atlas of Hematopathological Disease

Alan D. Ramsay
University College London Hospitals, London, UK

Manuel Rodriguez-Justo
University College London Hospitals, London, UK

Scott J. Rodig
Harvard Medical School, Brigham and Women's Hospital, Boston, Massachusetts, USA

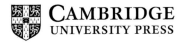

CAMBRIDGE
UNIVERSITY PRESS

CAMBRIDGE
UNIVERSITY PRESS

University Printing House, Cambridge CB2 8BS, United Kingdom

Published in the United States of America by Cambridge University Press, New York

Cambridge University Press is part of the University of Cambridge.

It furthers the University's mission by disseminating knowledge in the pursuit of education, learning and research at the highest international levels of excellence.

www.cambridge.org
Information on this title: www.cambridge.org/9781107624542

© Alan D. Ramsay, Manuel Rodriguez-Justo and Scott J. Rodig

First published 2014

Printed in Spain by Gratos SA, Arte sobre papel

A catalogue record for this publication is available from the British Library

ISBN 978-1-107-62454-2 (PACK/PB+CD)
ISBN 978-1-107-66115-8 (PB)
ISBN 978-1-107-65607-9 (CD)

Contents

Clinical utility of core biopsies   page vi
Christopher McNamara

1. **Reactive lymph nodes**   1
   Illustrative cases: Reactive lymph nodes   7

2. **Specific reactive conditions in lymph nodes**   12
   Illustrative cases: Specific reactive conditions in lymph nodes   30

3. **Classical Hodgkin lymphoma**   35
   Illustrative case: Classical Hodgkin lymphoma   40

4. **Nodular lymphocyte predominant Hodgkin lymphoma**   43
   Illustrative case: Nodular lymphocyte predominant Hodgkin lymphoma   49

5. **Follicular lymphoma**   52
   Illustrative cases: Follicular lymphoma   59

6. **Mantle cell lymphoma**   64
   Illustrative case: Mantle cell lymphoma   68

7. **Burkitt lymphoma**   71
   Illustrative case: Burkitt lymphoma   76

8. **Marginal zone lymphoma and lymphoplasmacytic lymphoma**   79
   Illustrative case: Marginal zone lymphoma and lymphoplasmacytic lymphoma   84

9. **Diffuse large B cell lymphoma**   87
   Illustrative cases: Diffuse large B cell lymphoma   96

10. **Chronic lymphocytic leukemia/small lymphocytic lymphoma**   105
    Illustrative case: Chronic lymphocytic leukemia/small lymphocytic lymphoma   109

11. **Lymphoblastic leukemia/lymphoma**   112
    Illustrative case: Lymphoblastic leukemia/lymphoma   117

12. **Nodal mature T cell lymphomas**   120
    Illustrative case: Nodal mature T cell lymphomas   131

13. **Plasma cell neoplasms**   134
    Illustrative cases: Plasma cell neoplasms   139

14. **Other pathology seen in lymph node needle core biopsies**   144
    Illustrative cases: Other pathology seen in lymph node needle core biopsies   155

Index   161

CD-ROM contains all figures from the book.

Clinical utility of core biopsies

Christopher McNamara Department of Haematology, The Royal Free Hospital, London

A tissue diagnosis by an expert hematopathologist is essential for all patients with suspected hematological malignancy for whom consideration of therapy is appropriate.[1] Treatment is increasingly specific and driven by protocol to optimize response and reduce toxicity; the emergence of new agents targeted to World Health Organization disease entities is likely to further underline the importance of an accurate diagnosis.

Traditionally, diagnosis of hematologic malignancy has been made by excision biopsy of an enlarged lymph node. In many circumstances this approach is problematic for several reasons. The lymph node in question may be located internally and require a prolonged and complicated surgical procedure to obtain access to it. The median age of onset of the two most common lymphoma subtypes affecting Western populations is in the seventh decade of life. Co-morbidities are frequently an issue, complicating general anesthesia and prolonged surgical times in this patient group. In addition, the delay required to organize such a procedure and the necessary recovery time from surgery mean that the initiation of myelosuppressive chemotherapy may need to be postponed. The effect of this on patient outcome is difficult to define; for patients with indolent lymphoma this may be irrelevant but it may be an important consideration for those with diseases that show an aggressive behavior. Finally, many patients, particularly those with lymphomas that have a high proliferation fraction and aggressive clinical behavior, will not be fit enough for a formal excision procedure due to disease burden.

There is evidence that many hemato-oncologists have changed their practice in response to these issues and now obtain tissue from lymph nodes utilizing a core biopsy technique under ultrasound or computerized tomography (CT) scan guidance. There are several reasons why this has come about. Interventional radiology has emerged as a distinct radiology sub-specialty, aided by high-quality imaging available for planning a safe approach to almost every bodily cavity. The complexity and scope of interventional radiology procedures has increased significantly in recent years; according to a recent Royal College of Radiology workforce report, interventional radiology has grown as a consequence of the demand and interests of the consultant colleagues in the hospitals in which they work (http://www.rcr.ac.uk/content.aspx?PageID=1562). These advances mean that radiologically guided core biopsies can now successfully obtain tissue samples from sites where a conventional excision biopsy would require invasive surgery. In some centers whilst the superficial palpable nodes are still excised by surgeons, retroperitoneal nodes and other deep nodes are routinely sampled by the interventional radiologists. Why might hemato-oncologists be increasingly requesting this approach? Access to this service is typically much faster than referral to an appropriate surgeon firstly for assessment and then, subsequently, for the procedure itself. Even when there is a dedicated surgeon attached to rapid access or "lump-and-bump" clinics there is frequently a delay in obtaining an operation date and time. It has been mentioned above that patient fitness is frequently a concern with a surgical procedure. In contrast, even the sickest patients are able to undergo an image-guided core biopsy procedure, provided they are able to follow instructions, even in the presence of a significant co-morbidity.[2] Finally, an image-guided procedure is generally preferred by patients to a general anesthetic and recovery from a formal procedure. Therefore the procedure adds clinical value to a service by obtaining the material for diagnosis rapidly and safely, allowing for prompt administration of chemotherapy and by improving the patient experience.

National guidelines now endorse the provision of core biopsy material for diagnosis, provided that the amount of tissue obtained is satisfactory, reflecting the fact that such documents must be pragmatic and reflect real, everyday working practice.[3] This recommendation is also aligned with those from North America where core needle biopsy is recommended as a viable alternative to excision, with similar emphasis on ensuring that adequate material is provided.[4] Further evidence that practice has changed at the national level comes from dialogue regarding the effect of changing biopsy practice on clinical research. Increasingly, therapy directed at the underlying variation in biology of the neoplasm is being applied to clinical study design.[5] Invariably, this involves gene expression profiling and the requirement for tissue additional to that needed by the hematopathologist for diagnostic purposes. This can be achieved when a whole lymph node is excised, but if only a single core of tissue is provided then there may be little tissue available at the end of diagnostic work-up for further studies. This has been discussed at the national level, as there are potential difficulties in completing this type of study unless an understanding of the change in practice can be assimilated into study design. Other countries have addressed this issue by obtaining consent from patients at the time of biopsy for extra cores to be taken for research purposes. Additional core biopsies are still likely to be more acceptable to patients than a formal surgical procedure, provided that patients can be assured that diagnostic accuracy is preserved with the less invasive procedure.

It is essential that hematopathologists respond to this change in working practice. This is a significant challenge; the hematopathologist's responsibility to provide an accurate diagnosis for the patient remains the same regardless of whether an excised lymph node or core biopsy is provided, despite the fact that the amount of tissue in the latter represents at least two orders of magnitude less than that in a biopsy obtained via excision (Dr Rudzinski, Birmingham Heartlands Hospital, personal communication). However, the literature discussed above supports the use of core biopsy from the point of accuracy of diagnosis and the issue may now be perceived as ensuring that the expertize to interpret core biopsies is disseminated to those who are part of multidisciplinary teams who are charged with reviewing such material.

Other potential difficulties with a change to core biopsy as opposed to excision biopsy include access to the available expertise within interventional radiology. There is also a theoretical risk of sampling error, though this may also occur with direct visualization of lymph nodes at the time of excision. The biopsy sample submitted by an inexperienced operator may be too small for adequate diagnosis providing insufficient overall architectural information for the pathologist and potentially limiting the material available for ancillary studies. A potential problem with core biopsies is an increase in instances where the pathologist is unable to render a definitive diagnosis and can only provide a differential diagnosis. In such cases clinico-pathological discussion is required to determine whether to carry out a second core biopsy or to proceed to formal excision. This problem can be minimized by obtaining adequate sized biopsies. In a series of 55 patients from the West of Scotland Cancer Centre, Loudon and colleagues compared the median length of core biopsies from patients with a secure, confirmed diagnosis and those from patients where the hematopathologist was unable to make a diagnosis and the patient had to undergo a second core biopsy or an excision biopsy. The median length in the diagnostic group was 17 mm compared with 5 mm in the non-diagnostic group.[6]

In conclusion, several factors aimed at improving the outcome and experience of hematology patients coupled with the fact that formalized, sub-specialty training curricula in interventional procedures now attracts large numbers of radiology trainees means that core biopsy is likely to remain a key part of the diagnostic process in this patient group. It allows for rapid diagnosis and early commencement of treatment, where appropriate, and justifies the effort of the hematopathology community to develop and disseminate expertise on interpretation of these samples.

References

1. Parker A, Bain B, Devereux S, et al. Best practice in lymphoma diagnosis and reporting. British Committee for Standards in Haematology (BCSH) Guideline. Available at: http://www.bcshguidelines.com/documents/Lymphoma_diagnosis_bcsh_042010.pdf

2. El-Sharkawi D, Ramsay A, Cwynarski K, et al. Clinico-pathologic characteristics of patients with hepatic lymphoma diagnosed using image-guided liver biopsy techniques. *Leuk Lymphoma* 2011;**52**:2130–2134.

3. McNamara C, Davies J, Dyer M, et al. Haemato-oncology Task Force of the British Committee for Standards in Haematology (BCSH); British Society for Haematology Committee. Guidelines on the investigation and management of follicular lymphoma. *Br J Haematol* 2012;**156**:446–467.

4. Amador-Ortiz C, Chen L, Hassan A, et al. Combined core needle biopsy and fine-needle aspiration with ancillary studies correlate highly with traditional techniques in the diagnosis of nodal-based lymphoma. *Am J Clin Pathol* 2011;**135**:516–524.

5. Dunleavy K, Pittaluga S, Czuczman MS, et al. Differential efficacy of bortezomib plus chemotherapy within molecular subtypes of diffuse large B-cell lymphoma. *Blood* 2009;**113**:6069–6076.

6. Loudon G, Kay D, Hilmi O, et al. Successful diagnosis of lymphoma from core biopsies. International Conference on Malignant Lymphoma (ICML), Lugano, June 2011. Abstract 394. Available at: http://www.lymphcon.ch/doc/ICML_AbstractBooks_vecchi/11-ICMLJune15-182011/68_Publication_Pathology-iv211-4.pdf

Reactive lymph nodes

Core biopsies from reactive lymph nodes are some of the more difficult specimens to interpret. These biopsies can contain multiple tissue compartments that include germinal centers, mantle zones, paracortex, sinuses, capsule, medulla and even hilum. The normal spatial organization is often distorted making morphological interpretation difficult. The pathological assessment of core biopsies from reactive nodes involves the active identification of a number of normal nodal compartments – the lymphoid follicles, the sinuses, the paracortex and the medulla.

Lymphoid follicles with germinal centers

The germinal center is the most important landmark in a reactive biopsy. Morphologically the germinal center contains collections of large centroblastic cells with a variable number of centrocytes interspersed with tingible body macrophages (Fig. 1.1A–D). The presence of a mantle zone composed of small mature lymphocytes will confirm the lymphoid follicle. Immunohistochemistry is key to the proper detection of germinal centers – the germinal centers in a reactive lymphoid follicle will express B lineage markers (Fig. 1.1E) and show up as mostly negative areas on CD3 (Fig. 1.1F). Reactive germinal center cells are both CD10 and bcl-6 positive and bcl-2 negative (Fig. 1.1G).[1,2] CD21 (and to a lesser extent CD23) will show underlying well-defined networks of follicular dendritic cells (FDCs) (Fig. 1.1H).[3] MIB1/Ki67 shows a high proliferation fraction within the germinal center[4] and ideally should identify normal germinal center light and dark zones (centrocyte-rich and centroblast-rich respectively),[5] although this zonation may not be prominent in core biopsies (Fig. 1.1I). The mantle zone B cells express IgD, IgM and bcl-2;[6] IgD is an excellent marker of mantle zones (Fig. 1.1J). CD3 will stain a variable number of T cells in the germinal centers (Fig. 1.1F). These T cells will be

bcl-2 positive and are follicular helper T cells, and so will also express CXCL13, ICOS and PD1.[7] There is often an accentuation of T cells at the periphery of the germinal center forming a vague rim below the mantle zone, which usually contains very few T cells and stands out as distinctly negative on CD3 staining. CD5 staining should resemble the pattern with CD3; expression of CD5 in the B cell areas of the node is indicative of lymphoma. Similarly cyclin D1, a marker of mantle cell lymphoma, should be negative in normal mantle zones.[8]

Lymphoid sinuses

The identification of sinuses in a core biopsy is often important in excluding a diagnosis of malignancy. Core biopsies may not contain the subcapsular sinus, but sinuses can frequently be seen in the specimen, and are evidence that the underlying architecture of the node is likely to be intact. Sinus boundaries may be poorly defined in core biopsies and, like germinal centers (see below), sinuses can show traumatic distortion and rupture (Fig. 1.1K,L). Morphologically the sinuses are less densely cellular than the rest of the node, and contain a variable mixture of histiocytes and small lymphocytes, with occasional larger transforming blasts. They are most easily recognized where there is sinus histiocytosis and numerous macrophages are present within the sinus spaces. Immunohistochemical identification is not usually required, but macrophage markers such as CD68, CD11c and CD163[9–11] can be used to identify collections of histiocytes within sinuses.

Paracortex

Morphologically the paracortical region is less well defined than the lymphoid follicles. There is a polymorphic cellular population containing small, medium and large-sized lymphocytes admixed with histiocytes, blood vessels with prominent endothelial

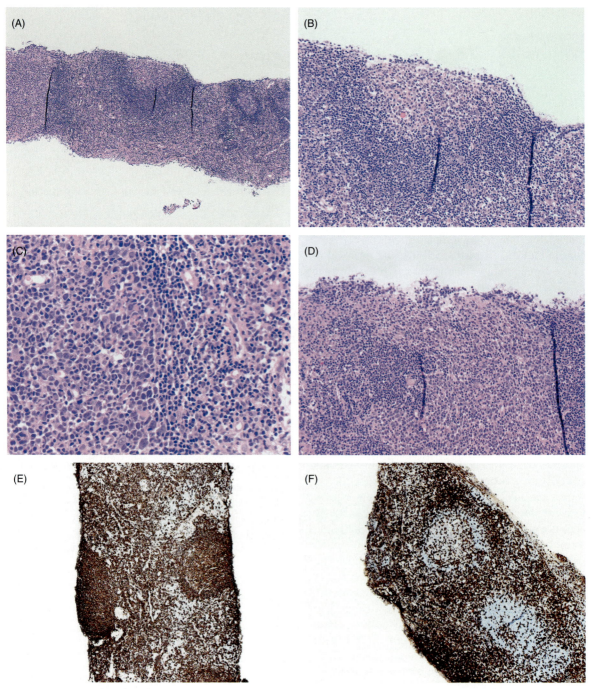

Figure 1.1 Reactive lymph node. (A,B) Low power H&E sections showing lymphoid follicles with germinal centers and mantle zones separated by the paracortex. (C) A high power view of a reactive germinal center containing a mixture of large nucleolated centroblastic cells and smaller centrocytes. The germinal center shows a well-defined edge and a thin mantle zone. Tingible body macrophages are not apparent in this image. (D) An enlarged and irregular germinal center with some distortion at the edge of the biopsy. (E) A CD20 stain highlighting the follicles and showing a moderate number of interfollicular B cells. (F) CD3 staining showing the interfollicular and intrafollicular T cells. (G) Bcl-2 staining that is negative in the reactive germinal center; the intrafollicular T cells and mantle zone cells are positive. (H) CD21 stain shows the follicular dendritic cell networks underlying the follicles. (I) MIB1 staining shows a high proliferation fraction in the germinal centers; clear zonation is rare in core biopsies. (J) An IgD stain that highlights the mantle zones. (K,L) H&E stains of lymphoid sinuses. The sinus is poorly defined and shows cellular distortion at the edge of the biopsy. The higher power view (L) shows a mixture of large pale histiocytes, small lymphocytes and scattered larger lymphoid cells. (M,N) Images from a biopsy showing paracortical hyperplasia. The paracortex is vascular and the blood vessels show prominent endothelial cells. Between the vessels there is a mixture of small, medium sized and large lymphocytes, and occasional eosinophils. (O) The large lymphoid cells are transforming B immunoblasts, and are positive with CD20. (P) An H&E stain of a distorted germinal center at the edge of a core biopsy. This peripheral "streaming" effect can be seen in CD10 (Q) and bcl-6 stains (R), both of which highlight the normal and distorted germinal centers.

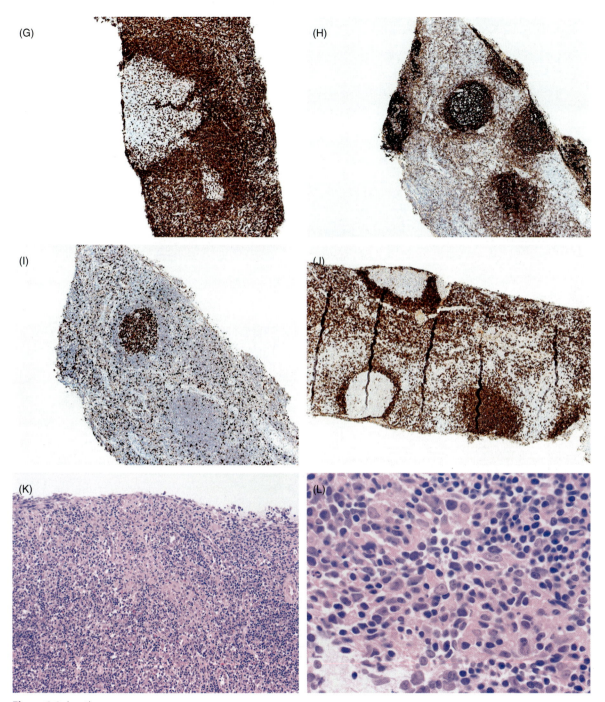

Figure 1.1 (cont.)

cells and occasional eosinophils and plasma cells (Fig. 1.1M–N). The lymphocytes are predominantly T cell and mark with CD3 and other pan-T cell markers (CD2, CD5 and CD7[12]). CD4 and CD8 show a mixture of helper and suppressor/cytotoxic subsets with a predominance of CD4-positive cells. Antigen-presenting cells (the interdigitating dendritic cells [IDCs]) are also present and are prominent in nodes showing a dermatopathic reaction. Langerhans cells are admixed with the IDCs, and the combined population

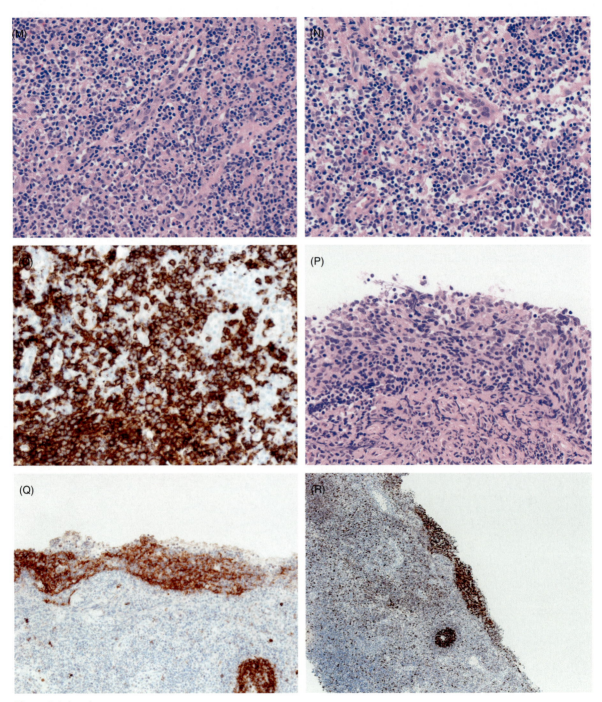

Figure 1.1 (cont.)

can be highlighted by CD1a and S100 staining.[13] The normal paracortical region will also contain a number of B cells. Amongst these are large transforming cells that have exited the germinal center and show immunoblastic morphology with a large nucleus and prominent central nucleolus (Fig. 1.1N,O). The proliferation fraction in the paracortex is variable, with MIB1/KI67 showing between 10 and 60% of cells in cycle.

Table 1.1 The main antibodies useful in the assessment of needle core biopsies from reactive lymph nodes

Antibody	Utility
CD20	Main B lineage marker
CD3	Main T lineage marker (also CD2, CD5, CD7)
CD10	Germinal center cells
Bcl-6	Germinal center cells
Bcl-2	Negative in germinal center cells in reactive follicles; positive in mantle zone B cells, T cells, plasma cells and most B cell lymphomas
CD21	Follicular dendritic cells (also CD23)
IgM, IgD	Mantle zone cells
Ki67/MIB1	Identifies the high proliferation fraction in germinal centers (with zonation)
CD5	T lineage marker that detects CD5-positive B cells in mantle cell lymphoma and chronic lymphocytic leukemia/small lymphocytic lymphoma
Cyclin D1	Useful for the exclusion of mantle cell lymphoma
CD138 (Syndecan)	Plasma cells

Medulla

Core biopsies in which the medulla is present can show collections of plasma cells and prominent sinuses, often with histiocytes. The plasma cells will be negative for CD20 and CD3 and will express CD138, CD38 and IRF4/MUM.[14] Light chain staining will be polytypic and Ki67/MIB1 will usually show a very low proliferation fraction (less than 10%) in this area.

Immunohistochemistry

Table 1.1 lists the main antibodies helpful in the pathological assessment of reactive lymph nodes in core biopsies.

Reactive nodes: problems and pitfalls of core biopsies

- A particular problem associated with core biopsy specimens is the traumatic distortion of germinal centers induced by the biopsy process. Affected germinal centers can be fragmented and compressed, with loss of nuclear morphology. Extreme cases show germinal centers stretched along the periphery of the core in a "streaming"

fashion. This peripheral streaming of germinal centers is not uncommon, and can be confirmed by CD10, bcl-6 and CD21 staining (Fig. 1.1P–R).
- Follicular lysis may make identification of germinal centers difficult, but use of IgD, CD21, CD10 and bcl-6 should clarify the situation. The mantle zone cells will be IgD positive and can be identified as a distinct population amongst the CD10 positive, bcl-6-positive germinal center cells.
- Primary follicles can also lead to some confusion – these will be composed of IgM-positive, IgD-positive, bcl-2-positive mantle zone cells and will have CD21-positive FDC networks. Germinal center cells will be absent, so CD10 and bcl-6 are negative, and MIB1/Ki67 will not show a high proliferation fraction.
- The presence of scattered large cells with immunoblastic features is normal in the paracortical region of reactive nodes. These will be a mixture of transforming T and B immunoblasts and should not be interpreted as malignant. These cells often express CD30; B immunoblasts will be IgM positive and should show polytypic light chain staining whereas the T immunoblasts should show both CD4 and CD8-positive subsets.

References

1. Dogan A, Bagdi E, Munson P, Isaacson PG. CD10 and BCL-6 expression in paraffin sections of normal lymphoid tissue and B-cell lymphomas. *Am J Surg Pathol* 2000;**24**:846–852.

2. Wang T, Lasota J, Hanau CA, Miettinen M. Bcl-2 oncoprotein is widespread in lymphoid tissue and lymphomas but its differential expression in benign versus malignant follicles and monocytoid B-cell proliferations is of diagnostic value. *APMIS* 1995;**103**:655–662.

3. Gloghini A, Carbone A. The nonlymphoid microenvironment of reactive follicles and lymphomas of follicular origin as defined by immunohistology on paraffin-embedded tissues. *Hum Pathol* 1993;**24**:67–76.

4. McCormick D, Chong H, Hobbs C, Datta C, Hall PA. Detection of the Ki-67 antigen in fixed and wax-embedded sections with the monoclonal antibody MIB1. *Histopathology* 1993;**22**:355–360.

5. MacLennan IC. Germinal centers. *Annu Rev Immunol* 1994;**12**:117–139.

6. Stein H, Bonk A, Tolksdorf G, et al. Immunohistologic analysis of the organization of normal lymphoid

tissue and non-Hodgkin's lymphomas. *J Histochem Cytochem* 1980;**28**:746–760.

7. Rodriguez-Justo M, Attygalle AD, Munson P, et al. Angioimmunoblastic T-cell lymphoma with hyperplastic germinal centres: a neoplasia with origin in the outer zone of the germinal centre? Clinicopathological and immunohistochemical study of 10 cases with follicular T-cell markers. *Mod Pathol* 2009;**22**:753–761.

8. Raffeld M, Sander CA, Yano T, Jaffe ES. Mantle cell lymphoma: an update. *Leuk Lymphoma* 1992;**8**:161–166.

9. Pulford KA, Sipos A, Cordell JL, Stross WP, Mason DY. Distribution of the CD68 macrophage/myeloid associated antigen. *Int Immunol* 1990;**2**:973–980.

10. Cabañas C, Sanchez-Madrid F, Acevedo A, et al. Characterization of a CD11c-reactive monoclonal

antibody (HC1/1) obtained by immunizing with phorbol ester differentiated U937 cells. *Hybridoma* 1988;**7**:167–176.

11. Lau SK, Chu PG, Weiss LM. CD163: a specific marker of macrophages in paraffin-embedded tissue samples. *Am J Clin Pathol* 2004;**122**:794–801.

12. Mason DY, Gatter KC. The role of immunocytochemistry in diagnostic pathology. *J Clin Pathol* 1987;**40**:1042–1054.

13. Shinzato M, Shamoto M, Hosokawa S, et al. Differentiation of Langerhans cells from interdigitating cells using CD1a and S-100 protein antibodies. *Biotech Histochem* 1995;**70**:114–118.

14. Natkunam Y, Warnke RA, Montgomery K, Falini B, van De Rijn M. Analysis of MUM1/IRF4 protein expression using tissue microarrays and immunohistochemistry. *Mod Pathol* 2001;**14**:686–694.

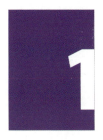

Illustrative cases: Reactive lymph nodes

Illustrative case 1

History: Female aged 45. Multiple enlarged axillary nodes; the referring pathologist could not rule out a "low grade lymphoma."

Comments: This is a case of HIV lymphadenopathy. The core biopsy contains follicles with an odd morphology; centroblasts are difficult to identify and the follicles have thin mantle zones. However there are well-defined T cell and B cell compartments and the phenotype of the germinal centers is normal (CD20 positive, CD10 positive, bcl-6 positive and bcl-2 negative). CD21 shows FDC networks, and staining for the p24 protein is positive on FDC confirming diagnosis of HIV lymphadenopathy.

It is rare to identify a specific cause for the changes seen in reactive lymph nodes. Lymph nodes from patients with HIV show a variety of pathological features. Germinal centers may be enlarged and irregular, or may be compact and dense, as seen here. Other potential findings include the presence of monocytoid B cells and a reactive plasmacytosis. P24 staining of the FDC networks is diagnostic.[1]

References

1. Baroni CD, Pezzella F, Mirolo M, Ruco LP, Rossi GB. Immunohistochemical demonstration of p24 HTLV III major core protein in different cell types within lymph nodes from patients with lymphadenopathy syndrome (LAS). *Histopathology* 1986;**10**:5–13.

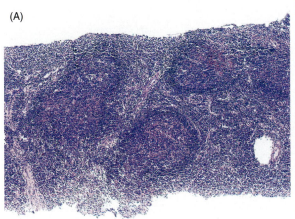
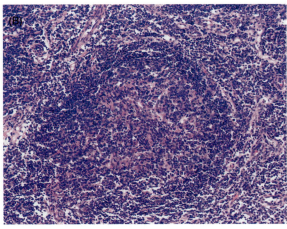

Illustrative case 1 (A–C) H&E stains showing germinal centers, mantle zones and paracortex. The follicles show poorly defined mantle zones and at high power lack identifiable centroblasts and tingible body macrophages. There is apparent extension of mantle zone cells into the germinal center. CD20 and CD3 (D,E) show B and T cell compartments (follicles and paracortex) and CD21 confirms follicular dendritic cell (FDC) networks (F). The germinal center cells are CD10 and bcl-6 positive (G,H) and show a high proliferation fraction with MIB1, with some zonation (I). Immunohistochemical staining for P24 protein (J) is positive on the FDC cells in the germinal centers, indicating human immunodeficiency virus (HIV) infection.

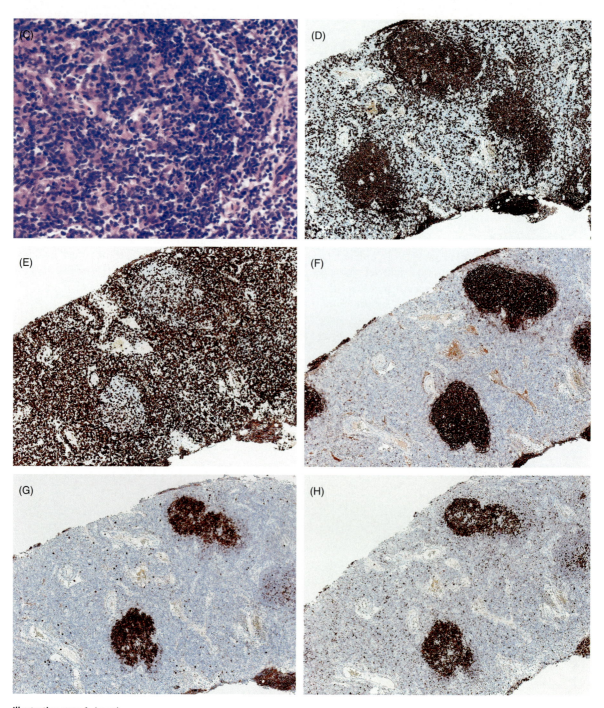

Illustrative case 1 (cont.)

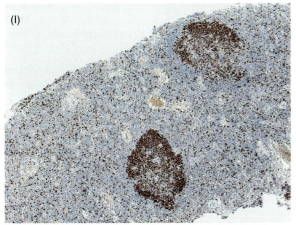
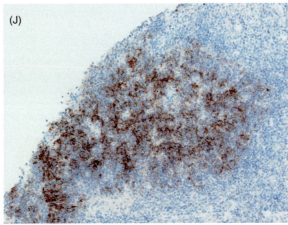

Illustrative case 1 (cont.)

Illustrative case 2

History: Female aged 48. Enlarged axillary lymph node. The referring pathologist made a diagnosis of follicular lymphoma based on "solid" follicles that were bcl-2 positive.

Comments: This case represents the pitfall of misinterpreting primary lymphoid follicles. The biopsy shows a follicular architecture and the follicles present are composed of monomorphic small lymphocytes. These lymphocytes express CD20 and bcl-2, and CD21 shows associated FDC networks. However, CD10 and bcl-6 are negative, so there are no germinal center cells present, and the small cells are IgD positive indicating a mantle zone phenotype. In addition the biopsy contains intact lymphoid sinuses and MIB1 shows almost no proliferation in the follicles.

Primary follicles lack germinal center cells and are composed of small lymphocytes with a mantle zone phenotype (CD20 positive, IgM positive, IgD positive, bcl-2 positive, CD10 negative and bcl-6 negative). They will show associated FDC networks with CD21 or CD23. The proliferation fraction will be very low (lower than most follicular lymphomas) and the nodal architecture will be preserved. Light chain staining will show a polytypic picture.

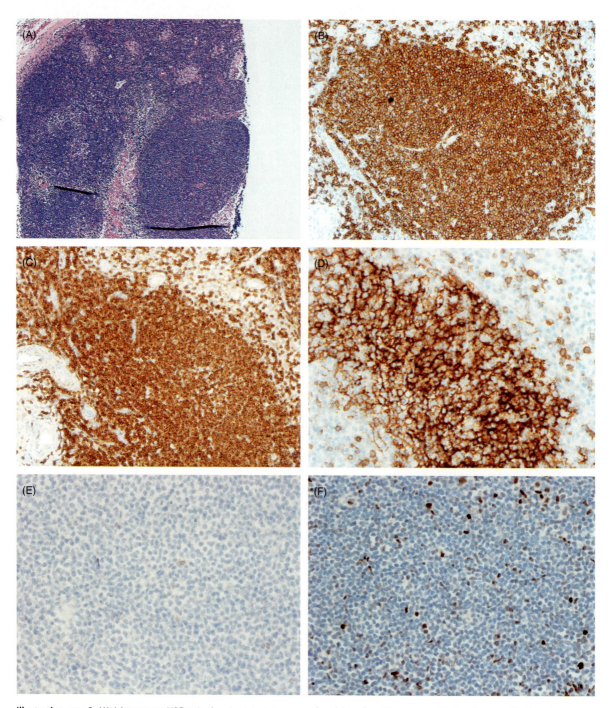

Illustrative case 2 (A) A low power H&E stain showing intact sinuses and nodules of small monomorphic lymphocytes. The lymphocytes are CD20-positive B cells (B) and are bcl-2 positive (C). The nodules show networks of follicular dendritic cells (FDCs) with CD21 (D), but CD10 and bcl-6 staining are negative (E,F). IgD staining (G) shows that the majority of cells in the nodules are mantle zone cells and MIB1 (H) shows an absence of proliferative activity.

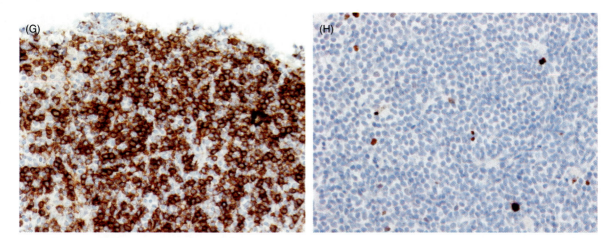

Illustrative case 2 (cont.)

Chapter 2

Specific reactive conditions in lymph nodes

Whilst many lymph core biopsies show reactive changes in which no specific underlying disease can be identified, there are a number of non-neoplastic conditions in which more specific diagnostic features are present. These conditions include, but are not limited to:

- Granulomatous disease – tuberculosis, sarcoid;
- Toxoplasmosis;
- Castleman disease (hyaline-vascular and plasma cell subtypes);
- Kikuchi lymphadenitis (KL; Kikuchi–Fujimoto disease);
- Infectious mononucleosis (IM);
- Dermatopathic lymphadenopathy.

Core biopsies may not be fully diagnostic in these conditions, but in many cases can raise a high degree of suspicion and can point the clinical teams towards the correct investigations required to confirm the underlying disease.

Tuberculosis

Core biopsy diagnosis of tuberculosis does not differ significantly from that of excision biopsies. The nodal architecture is partly or wholly destroyed by the presence of granulomas containing epithelioid macrophages with Langhans type giant cells and central caseous necrosis (Fig. 2.1A–C). The relatively small amount of tissue in core biopsies can make identification of large granulomas difficult, particularly if there is extensive caseation. In such specimens there may be more necrosis than viable lymphoid tissue, and the diagnosis may rest upon scattered clusters of epithelioid macrophages and occasional giant cells at the periphery of the necrotic areas (Fig. 2.1D,E). More chronic cases show fibrosis around the granulomas (Fig. 2.1F), adding further complexity to the diagnosis. Ziehl–Neelsen staining for acid-fast bacilli is usually performed (Fig. 2.1G), although very few cases contain detectable organisms. Polymerase chain reaction (PCR) for tuberculosis is also available,[1] but the results can be negative even in cases with otherwise typical pathology. Where there is extensive necrosis it is sometimes useful to carry out immunohistochemistry to try to exclude lymphoma. Sheets of necrotic B or T cells will often retain their lineage markers so extensive positivity should raise the suspicion of a lymphoma and lead to a request for repeat biopsy.[2]

Sarcoid

As with tuberculosis, the appearances on core biopsy resemble those seen in excision biopsies. The granulomas are usually small and well-defined, lack central caseation (although central necrosis can be seen) and should show foreign-body type rather than Langhans type giant cells, but in practice these two cell types show a significant morphological overlap (Fig. 2.2A–D). Fibrosis is more prominent in sarcoid than in tuberculosis, and the granulomas are often set in dense fibrous tissue (Fig. 2.2E,F). Some cases may show asteroid or Schaumann bodies within giant cells or granulomas.[3] Correlation with the clinical features is of critical importance in the diagnosis of sarcoidosis.

Toxoplasmosis

Core biopsy diagnosis of toxoplasmosis can be challenging. A triad of morphological features is typically required for the diagnosis:[4,5]

- Lymphoid follicles with enlarged, irregular ("geographic") germinal centers;
- Small (micro-) granulomas that are found within germinal centers;
- Monocytoid B cells in lymph node sinuses.

In practice the limited diameter of the core means that it can be difficult to assess germinal center enlargement and geographic outlines may not be apparent. The small granulomas within the paracortex, mantle zones and germinal centers (Fig. 2.3A–D) can also be subtle

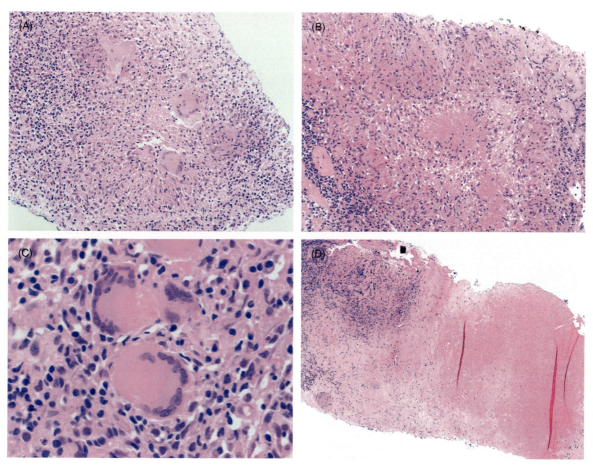

Figure 2.1 **Tuberculosis**. (A) An H&E stain of a typical tuberculous granuloma. There are epithelioid macrophages, Langhans' type giant cells and a small central area of caseation. (B) A case with more prominent caseation and fewer giant cells. Image (C) shows typical Langhans' type giant cell with the peripheral "horseshoe" arrangement of the nuclei. (D,E) A case with extensive caseous necrosis but only rare granulomas. (F) A case of tuberculosis (TB) with fibrotic granulomas. (G) A tuberculous granuloma negative for acid-fast bacteria (Ziehl–Neelsen stain).

and are easy to miss. Similarly, the collections of monocytoid B cells in the sinuses are rarely as obvious as they are in excision biopsies. The sinuses are often distorted and flattened, and the morphology of the monocytoid B cells is not as striking as in an excision (Fig. 2.3E). Although the diagnosis is essentially morphological, immunohistochemistry is very helpful in the confirmation of toxoplasmosis. The germinal center cells will be CD20 positive, CD10 positive, bcl-6 positive and bcl-2 negative and will show a high proliferation fraction with MIB1, sometimes with distinct zonation. These stains will enable a better assessment of the size and outline of the germinal centers than can be seen on H&E. Although the microgranulomas will express histiocytic markers such as CD68, CD11c (Fig. 2.3F) and CD163, the large number of background

macrophages in the lymph node can make small collections of histiocytes difficult to appreciate. However, the microgranulomas within the germinal centers will not express CD20, CD10, bcl-6 and MIB1 and so will stand out as "holes" with these stains (Fig. 2.3G,H). Additional staining with OCT-2, which marks germinal center cells and monocytoid B cells, is helpful (Fig. 2.3I).[6] OCT-2 positivity in sinuses, away from the germinal centers, will identify monocytoid B cells and confirm the final member of the morphological triad.

Castleman disease

The two forms of Castleman disease show different morphological features.[7] In the hyaline-vascular

13

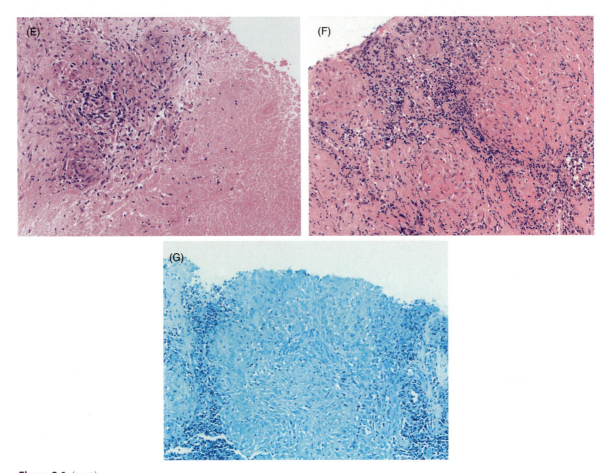

Figure 2.1 (cont.)

subtype the germinal centers are often small and show atrophic changes ("regressive transformation") with a reduction of germinal center B cells and an increase in follicular dendritic cells and blood vessels. The latter may show prominent endothelium, and a typical feature is the presence of blood vessels that extend from outside the lymphoid follicle, across the mantle zones and into the germinal center itself (the "tadpole" or "tennis racquet" sign). Mantle zones are expanded and the cells are often arranged in concentric rings ("onion-skinning"). The interfollicular zones are highly vascular, containing an irregular plexiform proliferation of small blood vessels with plump endothelial cells (Fig. 2.4A–C). Although primarily a morphological diagnosis, there are several immunohistochemical features that can help confirm the diagnosis. CD20 and CD3 show well-defined B cell and T cell compartments, and IgD stains cells in the expanded mantle zones (Fig. 2.4D–F). The germinal center cells are CD20 positive, CD10 positive, bcl-6 positive and bcl-2 negative with a high proliferation fraction. There may be gaps or holes in the germinal centers where the B cells are displaced by blood vessels (Fig. 2.4D). In many cases CD21 shows small, "tight" networks of follicular dendritic cells (FDCs) associated with atrophic follicles, and there can be focally expanded networks within which are two (or occasionally three) germinal centers ("twinning"). There are also fine concentric FDC networks associated with the "onion-skin" expanded mantle zones. The mantle zone cells express IgM and IgD, and CD123 shows a background increase in plasmacytoid dendritic cells within the interfollicular regions (Fig. 2.4G).[8] Plasma cells are rare in the paracortex and HHV8 staining is negative in this form of Castleman disease.

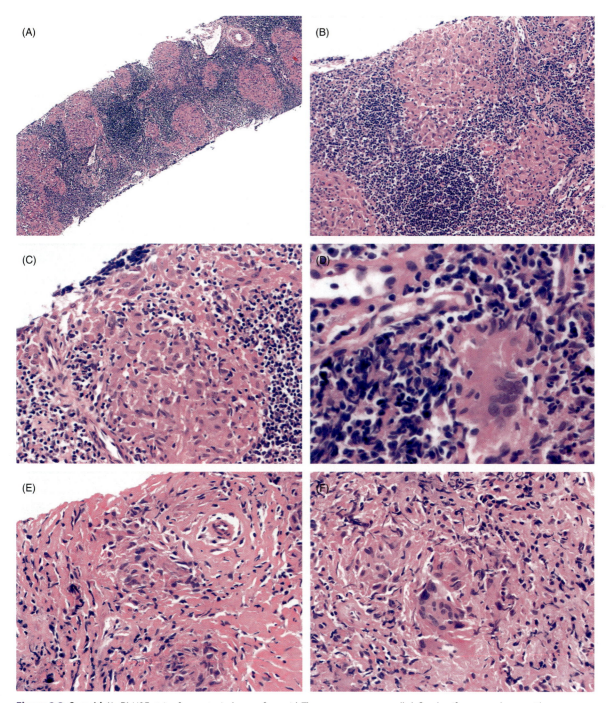

Figure 2.2 **Sarcoid**. (A–D) H&E stains from a typical case of sarcoid. There are numerous well-defined uniform granulomas with no evidence of caseation and no Langhans giant cells. The granulomas are made up of pale epithelioid cells (B,C) and occasional sarcoid giant cells are seen (D). (E,F) A case of sarcoid with extensive fibrosis; only a few small residual granulomas are present (F).

Plasma cell or multicentric Castleman disease is usually seen in the setting of human immunodeficiency virus (HIV), and is related to infection with Kaposi sarcoma (KS) virus (KSHV, HHV8). The germinal center changes are similar to those seen in hyaline-vascular Castleman disease, but may be less marked (Fig. 2.5A,B). The germinal centers are less atrophic, with a greater content of retained B cells,

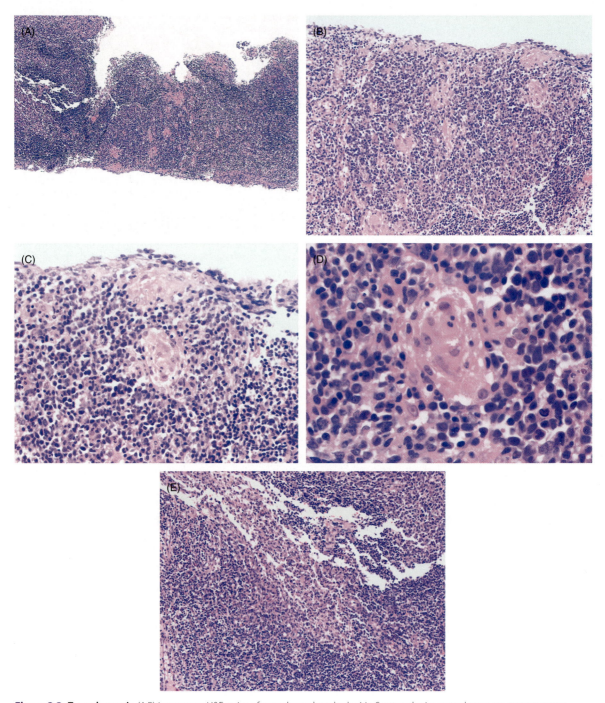

Figure 2.3 **Toxoplasmosis**. (A,B) Low power H&E stains of toxoplasma lymphadenitis. Scattered microgranulomas are present, many within germinal centers (B). Images (C,D) show higher power views of the toxoplasma microgranulomas. (E) A distorted lymph node sinus containing a collection of monocytoid B cells. (F) Microgranulomas in a germinal center stained with CD11c. (G,H) Images show "gaps" in bcl-6 and MIB1 staining in germinal centers due to the presence of the microgranulomas. (I) Sinusoidal monocytoid B cells express OCT-2.

and show more prominent penetration by blood vessels with plump endothelial cells. The concentric onion-skin mantle zone arrangement is also less marked than in the hyaline-vascular subtype. The interfollicular region contains blood vessels and sheets of mature plasma cells (Fig. 2.5C). A key feature is

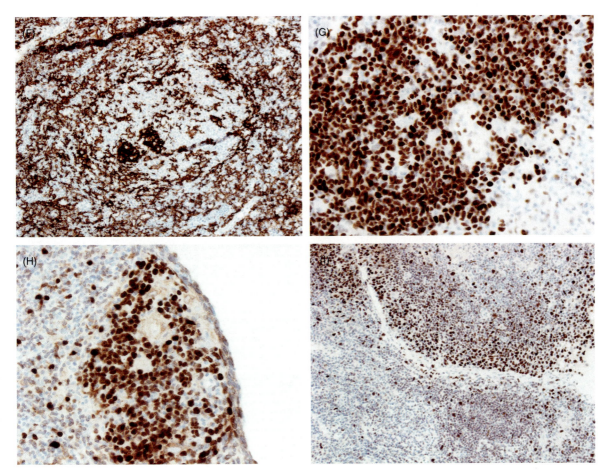

Figure 2.3 (cont.)

the presence of large plasmablastic cells at the periphery of the germinal centers, in the mantle zones and in the perifollicular region (Fig. 2.5D). Immunohistochemistry shows that these large cells are HHV8-positive, IgM-positive B cells, some with loss of CD20, and that they preferentially express lambda light chains although are not clonal (Fig. 2.5E–G).[9] The germinal center cells are CD20 positive, CD10 positive, bcl-6 positive and bcl-2 negative and MIB1 shows more activity than in hyaline-vascular Castleman disease. The FDC changes are also less prominent than in the hyaline-vascular subtype. The interfollicular plasma cells are CD138 positive (Fig. 2.5H) and show polytypic light chain staining. CD123 also shows increased plasmacytoid dendritic cells. In HIV patients there is a frequent association with KS, and HHV8 staining may show microscopic foci of KS within the biopsy.[10]

Kikuchi lymphadenitis (histiocytic necrotizing lymphadenitis)

In KL there are areas of intact nodal architecture and the paracortex contains abnormal foci composed of pale histiocytic cells and admixed lymphoid cells. More advanced disease shows central necrosis in these foci, but this is absent in the early (cellular) stage. Apoptosis is a feature at all stages and karyorrhectic nuclear debris is prominent in the abnormal cellular foci (Fig. 2.6A–C). The histiocytic cells show pale curved or crescentic nuclei and abundant eosinophilic cytoplasm (Fig. 2.6D,E). There is phagocytosis of the nuclear debris in many cells. Interspersed with these histiocytes are lymphoid cells, many with transformed "blastic" morphology. Neutrophils and plasma cells are typically absent. Towards the periphery of the abnormal foci and within the adjacent paracortex are medium-sized to large cells with hyperchromatic nuclei and basophilic

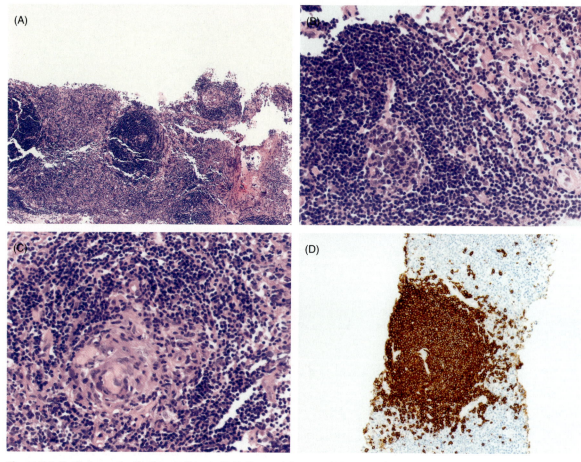

Figure 2.4 Hyaline-vascular Castleman disease. (A–C) Abnormal ("regressed") lymphoid follicles and vascular paracortex from a case of hyaline-vascular Castleman disease. There is some "hyaline" sclerosis in the paracortex (B), and expanded mantle zones (A,B). Occasional small blood vessels are seen to traverse the mantle zones (B). In the regressed germinal centers the germinal center cells are largely replaced by blood vessels and follicular dendritic cells (C). Image (D) is a CD20 stain showing a well-defined B cell follicle with an unstained prominent blood vessel. The surrounding paracortical region contains CD3-positive T cells (E). IgD staining (F) highlights expanded mantle zones around regressed germinal centers and CD123 staining (G) shows an increased number of CD123-positive plasmacytoid dendritic cells within the paracortex.

cytoplasm – the plasmacytoid dendritic cells. Kikuchi lymphadenitis is primarily diagnosed on the morphological features, but immunohistochemical confirmation is very helpful. The necrotic and proliferative appearance of the abnormal foci can be mistaken for a neoplastic proliferation (usually a T cell lymphoma); on occasion a malignant lymphoma with prominent apoptosis is mistakenly diagnosed as KL. The key features in identifying KL are:[11]

- Focal disease, with intact architecture outwith the abnormal areas.
- Apoptotic debris and an absence of neutrophils in the abnormal foci, whether or not there is necrosis.

- High content of histiocytes in the abnormal foci – CD11c positive, CD68 positive, CD163 positive, CD20 negative (Fig. 2.6F).
- Myeloperoxidase positivity in a subset of the histiocytes – granular cytoplasmic staining (Fig. 2.6G).[12]
- CD123 showing plasmacytoid dendritic cells within the necrotic foci and in the surrounding node (Fig. 2.6H).[13]
- Admixed T cells in the abnormal foci (Fig. 2.6I). These are transforming T immunoblasts and are predominantly CD8 positive; they also express cytotoxic markers (granzyme B, perforin, TIA1). There is a paucity of CD4-positive T cells in these areas.[14]

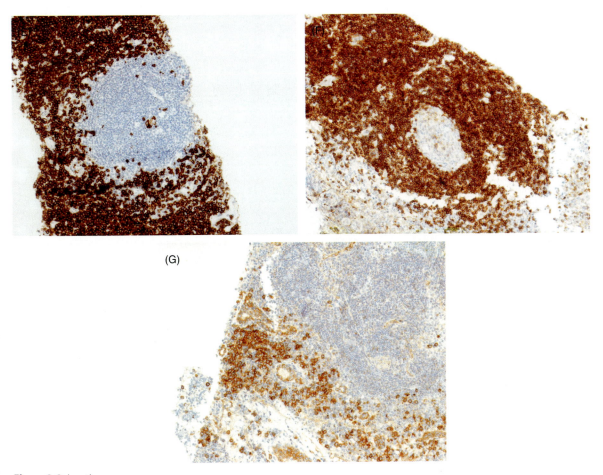

Figure 2.4 (cont.)

- MIB1 showing a high proliferation fraction (70–80%) in the involved areas.[14]

Kikuchi lymphadenitis is a self-limited condition, and can progress to a fibrous stage, so older cases may show non-specific changes. The literature indicates that lupus erythematosus can show identical histological features to KL.

Infectious mononucleosis

The lymph node changes seen in infectious mononucleosis (IM) may look extremely worrying in needle core biopsies, particularly where the clinical history supplied does not suggest an acute infectious process. Infection with the Epstein–Barr virus (EBV) leads to a marked proliferation of both B and T lymphoid cells.[15] Lymph nodes in IM show a preservation of the normal architecture and contain enlarged lymphoid follicles with reactive germinal centers in combination with an expanded and cellular paracortex. The germinal centers are composed predominantly of centroblasts and tingible body macrophages contain prominent nuclear debris. Mantle zones may be widened. The paracortex contains a polymorphic population of cells which includes a large number of transformed immunoblasts admixed with small lymphocytes, plasmacytic cells and histiocytes on a vascular background. The immunoblasts present show rounded nuclei with prominent nucleoli and prominent cytoplasm. Some of the immunoblasts can resemble mononuclear Hodgkin cells, suggesting a diagnosis of interfollicular classical Hodgkin lymphoma. Mitoses are frequent and the high concentration of transforming blast cells can resemble a large cell lymphoma such as diffuse large B cell lymphoma or anaplastic large cell lymphoma. A lymphoma diagnosis is more likely to be considered where the core consists mainly of

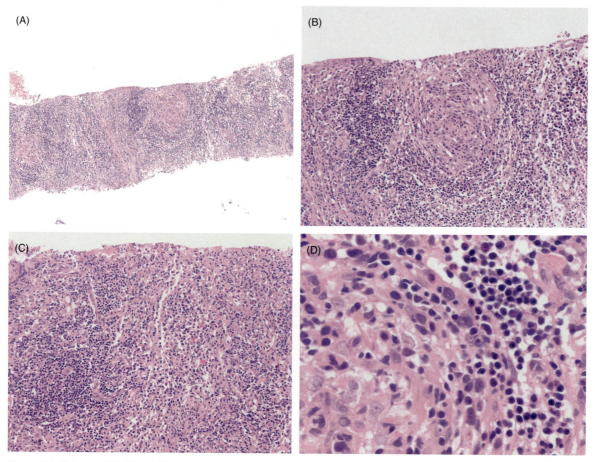

Figure 2.5 **Plasma cell Castleman disease**. (A) Low power H&E from a case of plasma cell Castleman disease in a human immunodeficiency virus (HIV) -positive patient. An abnormal follicle is present and prominent blood vessels are seen in the paracortex and crossing the mantle zone. (B) A regressed follicle with loss of germinal center cells and a blood vessel crossing the mantle to form the "tadpole" sign. The paracortical region is vascular and contains collections of plasma cells (C). At the periphery of the germinal centers there are large nucleolated plasmablasts (D). These plasmablasts stain positively for HHV8 (LANA) (E) and IgM (F) and show cytoplasmic expression of lambda light chains (G). The paracortical plasma cells are CD138 positive (H).

paracortical tissue, so that it is difficult or impossible to confirm an intact nodal architecture. Diagnostic clues to a diagnosis of IM include:

- Underlying nodal architecture remains intact.
- Germinal centers (where present) show reactive changes.
- Polymorphic immunoblast-rich paracortex with frequent mitoses (Fig. 2.7A–D).
- Transforming B and T cells in the paracortex, with a high proliferation fraction and expression of CD30 and MUM1 (Fig. 2.7E–G).
- Large paracortical B cells may show heterogeneous staining with CD20.
- Plasmacytic background population in the paracortex.

- EBER positivity in large and small B cells (Fig. 2.7H).[16]
- Polytypic light chain staining in B immunoblasts and in plasma cells (Fig. 2.7I,J).
- Paracortical T cell immunoblasts are predominantly CD8 positive and express cytotoxic markers (perforin, granzyme B, TIA-1).[17]
- PCR shows a polyclonal pattern (although oligoclonal and clonal populations can be detected in EBV infection[18]).

Dermatopathic lymphadenopathy

Where lymph nodes are draining skin-based disease the core biopsy may show specific changes in the

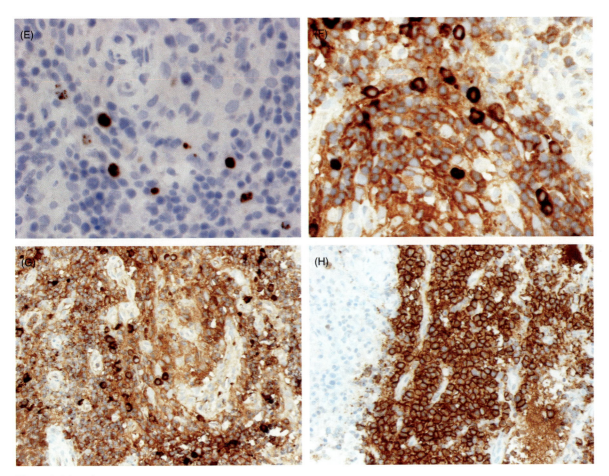

Figure 2.5 (cont.)

paracortex.[19] Many of the changes resemble those seen in non-specific paracortical hyperplasia, but in advanced disease the expanded paracortex can take on a nodular configuration, with B follicles either compressed between these nodules or even absent from the biopsy. At low power the nodules of expanded paracortex can show a form of "starry sky" pattern with prominent histiocytes and interdigitating dendritic cells giving the appearance of pale "stars" on a background of small lymphocytes (Fig. 2.8A,B). Although distorted, the underlying nodal architecture remains intact, and remaining normal sinuses may be present (Fig. 2.8C). At higher power a variable number of the histiocytes will contain granular melanin pigment in their cytoplasm (Fig. 2.8D). If immunohistochemistry is required, the small lymphocytes are CD3 positive and the majority are CD4 positive (Fig. 2.8E–G). CD20 shows the B cell areas between the paracortical

nodules. The expanded network of interdigitating dendritic cells can be demonstrated by CD1a and S100 staining (Fig. 2.8H, I).

Immunohistochemistry panel for specific non-neoplastic conditions

Table 2.1 lists an extended panel of antibodies useful in the diagnosis of specific non-neoplastic conditions in needle core biopsies of lymph nodes.

Problems and pitfalls of core biopsies in specific non-neoplastic conditions

The main problems in the core biopsy diagnosis of specific non-neoplastic conditions include:

- Limited tissue sampling. This affects many of the entities in this group. Tuberculous granulomas can

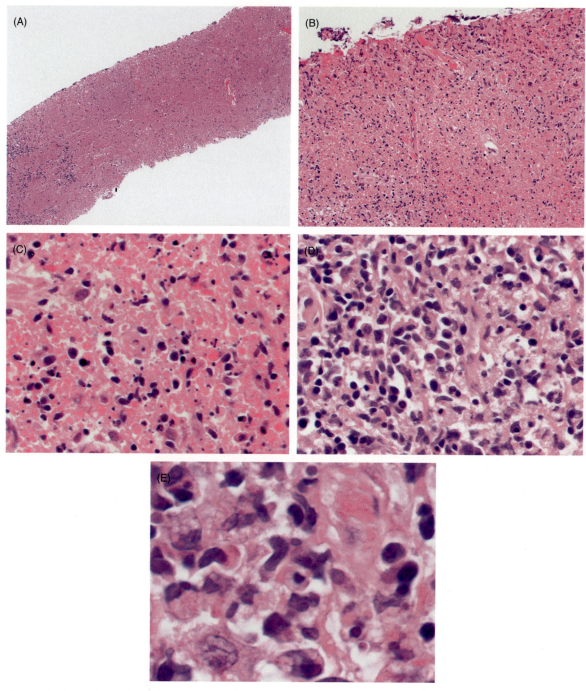

Figure 2.6 **Kikuchi lymphadenitis (KL)**. (A–C) H&E stains from the necrotic areas in a core biopsy from a case of KL. (C) A high power view showing hyperchromatic nuclei and characteristic apoptotic debris with an absence of neutrophils. Image (D) is from a non-necrotic, more cellular area and shows a mixture of histiocytic cells, plasmacytoid dendritic cells and lymphocytes. The histiocytes show pale, comma-shaped nuclei (E), and stain with CD11c (F). A sub-population of the histiocytes present show granular cytoplasmic staining with myeloperoxidase (G). The plasmacytoid dendritic cells are CD123 positive (H) and the T cells, many of which are transforming, are CD3 positive (I).

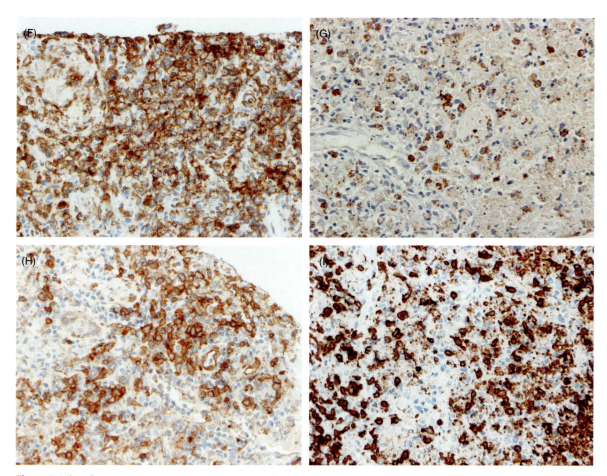

Figure 2.6 (cont.)

be difficult to define in a small biopsy, particularly where necrosis is extensive. Similarly KL can show extensive necrosis and so may lack identifiable features. In IM, reactive germinal centers may be few or even absent, suggesting architectural effacement and leading to a possible diagnosis of malignancy. Similarly the localization of dermatopathic changes to the paracortex may not be apparent and T cell lymphoma may be suspected.

- Tissue distortion in core biopsies. The traumatic effects of the biopsy process on the underlying architecture can interfere with the morphological features in many of these conditions. Specifically disruption may preclude the detection of microgranulomas within germinal centers, or monocytoid B cells in lymphoid sinuses.

- Morphological overlap. The primary diagnostic clues for many of the conditions in this group are morphological, and the pathologist has to recognize the possibility of a disease in order to request appropriate confirmatory immunohistochemistry. However, some of these specific reactive conditions can show a degree of morphological overlap, which is often more of a problem in core biopsies than in lymph node excisions. Tuberculosis and sarcoid may be impossible to distinguish when there are only a few scattered granulomas and non-specific giant cells with some background fibrosis. In this

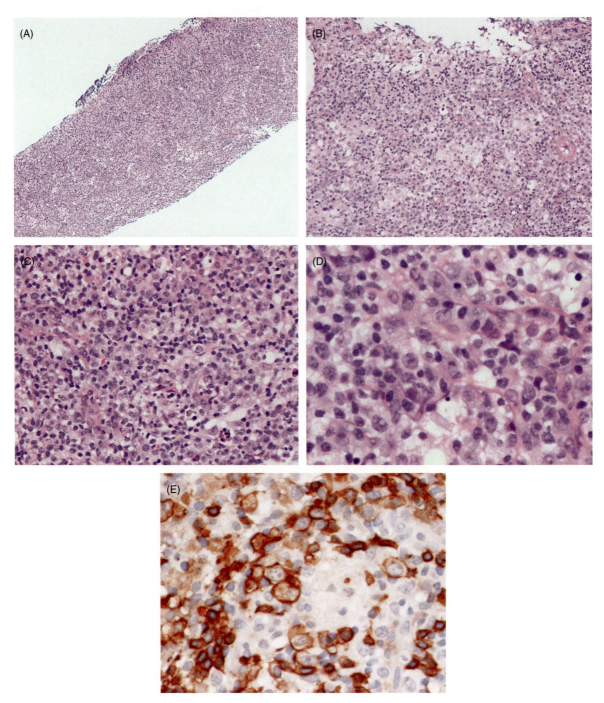

Figure 2.7 **Infectious mononucleosis**. (A–D) Images show the paracortical cellular infiltrate in a core biopsy from a case of infectious mononucleosis. The infiltrate is polymorphic, containing histiocytes, small lymphocytes and large transforming immunoblasts with prominent nucleoli. CD20 (E) identifies large B immunoblasts and CD3 (F) shows admixed large T immunoblasts. MIB1 shows a high proliferation fraction (G) and EBER in-situ hybridization is positive in both large and small cells (H). The large transforming B cells present show polytypic light chain staining (kappa is shown in I and lambda in J).

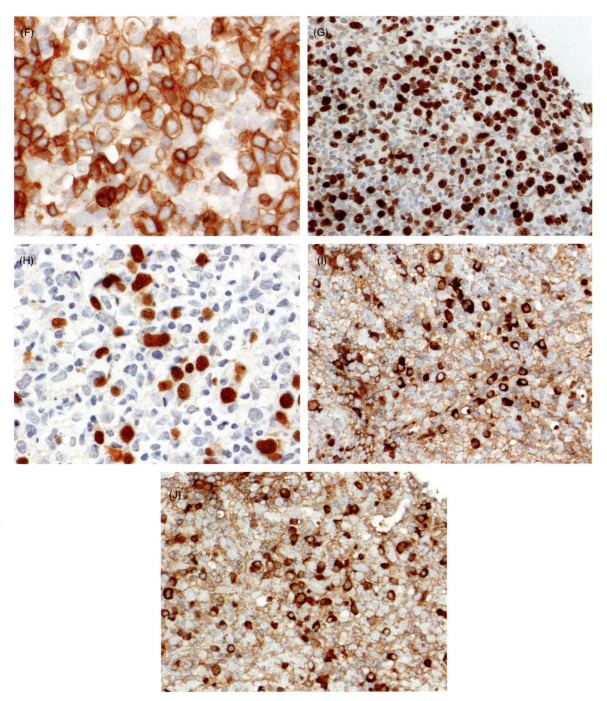

Figure 2.7 (cont.)

setting the clinical features may be more important than the pathology. Similarly hyaline-vascular and plasma cell Castleman disease can be difficult to separate on morphology alone; plasma cells are present in the hyaline-vascular subtype and prominent blood vessels are seen in plasma cell Castleman disease. Here the inclusion of HHV8 immunohistochemistry is critical.

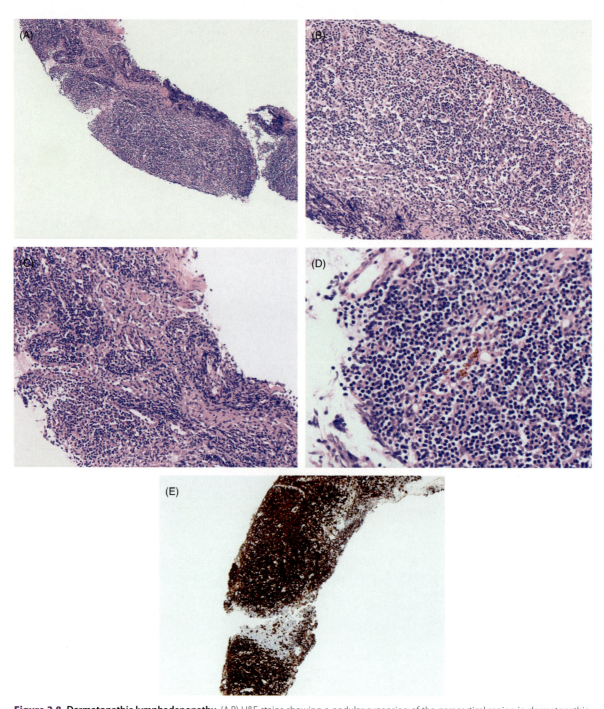

Figure 2.8 Dermatopathic lymphadenopathy. (A,B) H&E stains showing a nodular expansion of the paracortical region in dermatopathic lymphadenopathy. (C) Image shows intact sinuses. (D) A higher power view of the characteristic melanin-containing histiocytes in the expanded paracortex. Image (E) shows CD3 staining; most of the T cells present are CD4 positive (F), although CD8-positive cells are also present (G). Paracortical interdigitating dendritic cells can be highlighted with CD1a (H) or S100 (I).

- Sarcoid-like granulomas associated with lymphoma. Granulomatous inflammation resembling sarcoid or even tuberculosis can be seen in association with a number of lymphoid malignancies, in particular classical Hodgkin lymphoma. When granulomas are seen careful

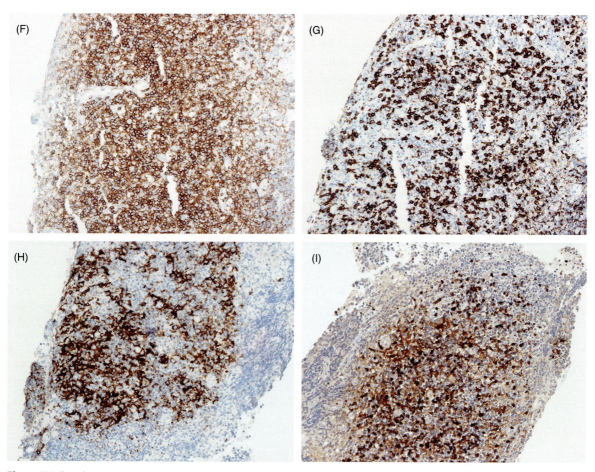

Figure 2.8 (cont.)

examination of the background lymphoid tissue is required to look for Hodgkin/Reed–Sternberg cells, pleomorphic lymphoid cells or a suspiciously monomorphic population. The presence of eosinophils is often a clue that should alert the pathologist to the possibility of classical Hodgkin lymphoma.

- High proliferation fractions. A number of the specific reactive conditions can show a high proliferation fraction with Ki67/MIB1 staining – IM, toxoplasmosis, KL. This should not form the basis of a diagnosis of malignancy. Pathologists are used to seeing high proliferation fractions in reactive germinal centers but can become worried when other parts of the node show this feature. One of the authors (AR) has

received a number of cases of KL with a diagnosis of T cell lymphoma, and also had considered a diagnosis of anaplastic large cell lymphoma in a case that turned out to be IM with proliferating large reactive T cells. Another biopsy was received where a diagnosis of toxoplasmosis was "excluded" due to a high proliferation rate. Ki67/MIB1 should be interpreted very carefully, taking into account the areas of the node affected, the possible conditions considered and the full clinical history. The pathologist should not hesitate to ask for ancillary tests (EBV serology, toxoplasma serology) from the clinical teams looking after the patient. Ki67/MIB1 staining alone is a very poor tool for identifying malignant disease.

Table 2.1 Extended table of antibodies used in the diagnosis of specific reactive conditions in lymph node core biopsies

Antibody	Condition	Utility
CD20	Various – general marker	Main B lineage marker
CD3	Various – general marker	Main T lineage marker (also CD2, CD5, CD7)
CD5	Various – general marker	T lineage marker useful in the exclusion of CD5-positive B cell neoplasms
CD10	Various – general marker	Germinal center cells
Bcl-6	Various – general marker	Germinal center cells
Bcl-2	Various – general marker	Negative in germinal center cells in reactive follicles; positive in mantle zone B cells, T cells, plasma cells and most B cell lymphomas
CD21	Various – general marker	Follicular dendritic cells (also CD23)
Ki67/MIB1	Various – general marker	Identifies the high proliferation fraction in germinal centers (with zonation)
MPO	KL	Granular cytoplasmic positivity in a sub-population of macrophages
CD123	KL, Castleman disease	Identifies plasmacytoid dendritic cells in KL and in Castleman disease
CD4, CD8	KL, IM	T subset markers. The necrotic areas in KL contain numerous transforming CD8-positive cells, and very few CD4-positive cells. In IM the paracortex also contains numerous transforming CD8-positive cells.
Perforin, TIA-1, granzyme B,	KL, IM	Cytotoxic markers. The transforming CD8 blasts in KL and IM strongly express these markers
S100	Dermatopathic lymphadenopathy	Stains interdigitating dendritic cells in the paracortex
CD1a	Dermatopathic lymphadenopathy	Stains interdigitating dendritic cells in the paracortex
HHV8 (LANA)	Plasma cell Castleman disease	Identifies HHV8 (KSHV) infected plasmablasts in plasma cell Castleman disease. Can also reveal microscopic Kaposi sarcoma
EBER	IM	Identifies EBV-infected B cells in infectious mononucleosis
OCT-2	Toxoplasmosis	Marks monocytoid B cells in sinuses (also positive in germinal center cells)
CD11c	Tuberculosis, sarcoid, toxoplasmosis, KL	Macrophage marker useful in identification of granulomas and histiocytes
CD68	Tuberculosis, sarcoid, toxoplasmosis, KL	Macrophage marker useful in identification of granulomas and histiocytes
CD163	Tuberculosis, sarcoid, toxoplasmosis, KL	Macrophage marker useful in identification of granulomas and histiocytes

Abbreviations: EBV, Epstein–Barr virus; IM, infectious mononucleosis; KL, Kikuchi lymphadenitis.

References

1. Ghossein RA, Ross DG, Salomon RN, Rabson AR. Rapid detection and species identification of mycobacteria in paraffin-embedded tissues by polymerase chain reaction. *Diagn Mol Pathol* 1992;**1**:185–191.

2. Norton AJ, Ramsay AD, Isaacson PG. Antigen preservation in infarcted lymphoid tissue. A novel approach to the infarcted lymph node using monoclonal antibodies effective in routinely processed tissues. *Am J Surg Pathol* 1988;**12**:759–767.

3. Hsu RM, Connors AF Jr, Tomashefski JF Jr. Histologic, microbiologic, and clinical correlates of the diagnosis of sarcoidosis by transbronchial biopsy. *Arch Pathol Lab Med* 1996;**120**:364–368.

4. Stansfeld AG. The histological diagnosis of toxoplasmic lymphadenitis. *J Clin Pathol* 1961;**14**:565–573.

5. Lin MH, Kuo TT. Specificity of the histopathological triad for the diagnosis of toxoplasmic lymphadenitis: polymerase chain reaction study. *Pathol Int* 2001;**51**:619–623.

6. Loddenkemper C, Anagnostopoulos I, Hummel M, et al. Differential Emu enhancer activity and expression of BOB.1/OBF.1, Oct2, PU.1, and immunoglobulin in reactive B-cell populations, B-cell non-Hodgkin lymphomas, and Hodgkin lymphomas. *J Pathol* 2004;**202**:60–69.

7. Palestro G, Turrini F, Pagano M, Chiusa L. Castleman's disease. *Adv Clin Path* 1999;**3**:11–22.

8. Rollins-Raval MA, Marafioti T, Swerdlow SH, Roth CG. The number and growth pattern of plasmacytoid dendritic cells vary in different types of reactive lymph nodes: an immunohistochemical study. *Hum Pathol* 2013;**44**:1003–1010.

9. Chadburn A, Hyjek EM, Tam W, et al. Immunophenotypic analysis of the Kaposi sarcoma herpesvirus (KSHV; HHV-8) -infected B cells in HIV$^+$ multicentric Castleman disease (MCD). *Histopathology* 2008;**53**:513–524.

10. Naresh KN, Rice AJ, Bower M. Lymph nodes involved by multicentric Castleman disease among HIV-positive individuals are often involved by Kaposi sarcoma. *Am J Surg Pathol* 2008;**32**:1006–1012.

11. Hutchinson CB, Wang E. Kikuchi–Fujimoto disease. *Arch Pathol Lab Med* 2010;**134**:289–293.

12. Pileri SA, Facchetti F, Ascani S, et al. Myeloperoxidase expression by histiocytes in Kikuchi's and Kikuchi-like lymphadenopathy. *Am J Pathol* 2001;**159**:915–924.

13. Kishimoto K, Tate G, Kitamura T, Kojima M, Mitsuya T. Cytologic features and frequency of plasmacytoid dendritic cells in the lymph nodes of patients with histiocytic necrotizing lymphadenitis (Kikuchi–Fujimoto disease). *Diagn Cytopathol* 2010;**38**:521–526.

14. Ohshima K, Kikuchi M, Sumiyoshi Y, et al. Proliferating cells in histiocytic necrotizing lymphadenitis. *Virchows Arch B Cell Pathol Incl Mol Pathol* 1991;**61**:97–100.

15. Ramsay AD. Reactive lymph nodes in pediatric practice. *Am J Clin Pathol* 2004;**122** Suppl:S87–97.

16. Hamilton-Dutoit SJ, Pallesen G. Detection of Epstein–Barr virus small RNAs in routine paraffin sections using non-isotopic RNA/RNA in situ hybridization. *Histopathology* 1994;**25**:101–111.

17. Williams ML, Loughran TP Jr, Kidd PG, Starkebaum GA. Polyclonal proliferation of activated suppressor/cytotoxic T cells with transient depression of natural killer cell function in acute infectious mononucleosis. *Clin Exp Immunol* 1989;**77**:71–76.

18. Gaillard F, Mechinaud-Lacroix F, Papin S, et al. Primary Epstein–Barr virus infection with clonal T-cell lymphoproliferation. *Am J Clin Pathol* 1992;**98**:324–333.

19. Good DJ, Gascoyne RD. Atypical lymphoid hyperplasia mimicking lymphoma. *Hematol Oncol Clin North Am* 2009;**23**:729–745.

2 Illustrative cases: Specific reactive conditions in lymph nodes

Illustrative case 1

History: Female aged 34. Cervical lymphadenopathy. Biopsy to exclude classical Hodgkin lymphoma.

Comments: This core biopsy shows no identifiable lymphoid follicles and an expanded paracortex. Within the paracortex there are small focal areas of necrosis with associated apoptosis and collections of pale histiocytes. Immunohistochemistry confirms a mixture of histiocytes, plasmacytoid dendritic cells and T cells. There is granular myeloperoxidase positivity in a sub-population of the histiocytes and the T cells are predominantly CD8 positive. The appearances are those of Kikuchi lymphadenitis.

The histology of Kikuchi lymphadenitis is quite variable, and not all cases have the typical clinical or pathological picture. Necrotic foci can be very small, but the presence of apoptosis should raise the possibility of Kikuchi lymphadenitis and a full immunohistochemical profile (see Table 2.1) will enable a positive diagnosis.

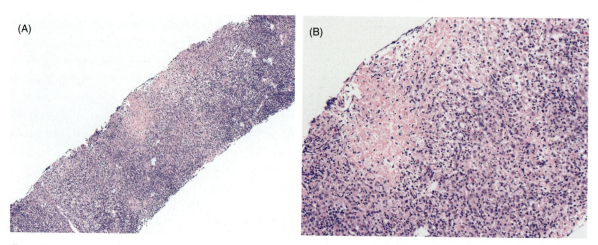

Illustrative case 1 The low power H&E stain (A) shows a small focus of necrosis in a biopsy consisting mainly of paracortex. At higher power (B,C) the necrotic area contains histiocytes and apoptotic debris, with an absence of neutrophils. In areas where there is less necrosis (pre-necrotic regions) there are sheets of foamy histiocytes with apoptotic debris (D,E). High power views of the cellular areas (F,G) show mixture of histiocytes, transforming lymphocytes, plasmacytoid dendritic cells and apoptotic bodies. Immunohistochemistry shows MPO-positive histiocytes in the necrotic areas (H). In the more cellular regions the sheets of histiocytes are CD11c positive (I), with admixed CD123-positive plasmacytoid dendritic cells (J) and CD8-positive T cells (K).

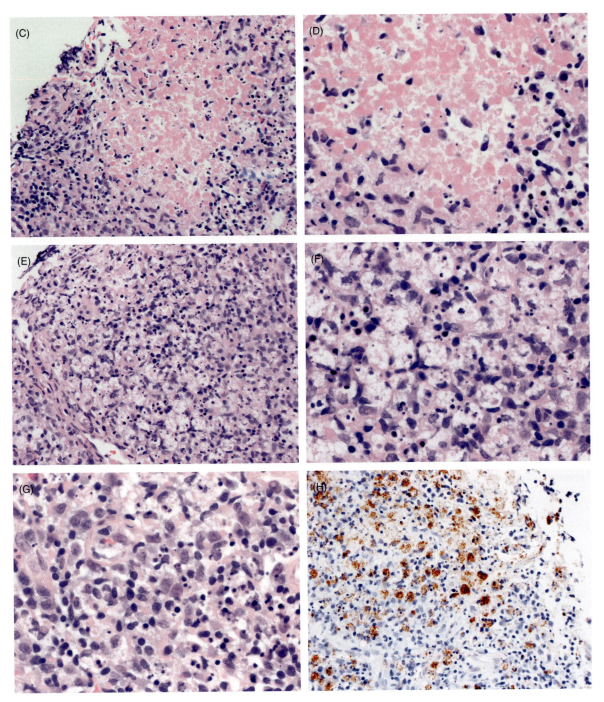

Illustrative case 1 (cont.)

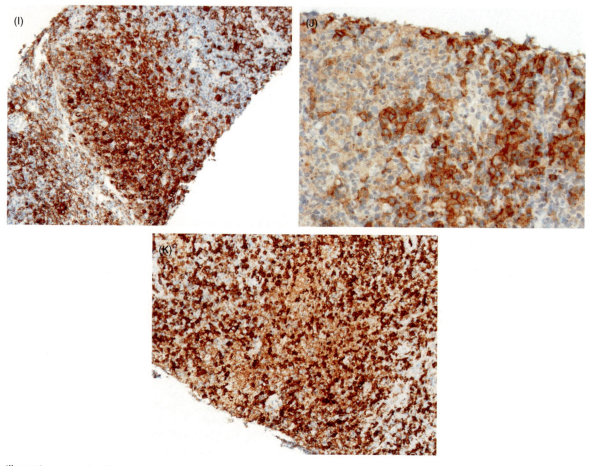

Illustrative case 1 (cont.)

Illustrative case 2

History: Female aged 42. Human immunodeficiency virus (HIV)-positive with decreased CD4 count. Pyrexia with axillary and retroperitoneal lymphadenopathy. Biopsy of retroperitoneal lymph node.

Comments: This is a short core biopsy showing little residual lymph node together with some fibrous tissue and collections of inflammatory cells. The appearances suggest an abscess and raise the possibility of a conventional bacterial infection. However, at the edge of the acute inflammation there are epithelioid macrophages and Ziehl–Neelsen staining shows the presence of frequent acid-fast bacteria.

Tuberculosis does not always show the typical histological pattern, particularly in the setting of HIV. Whilst Ziehl–Neelsen staining may rarely be positive in everyday practice in Western Europe and the USA, in HIV-positive patients it is a critical investigation, detecting disease that may not be clinically apparent or revealing the presence of non-reactive tuberculosis. This patient was also thought to suffer from plasma cell Castleman disease, but there was no nodal tissue in the biopsy to show the typical histological changes, and HHV8 staining was negative.

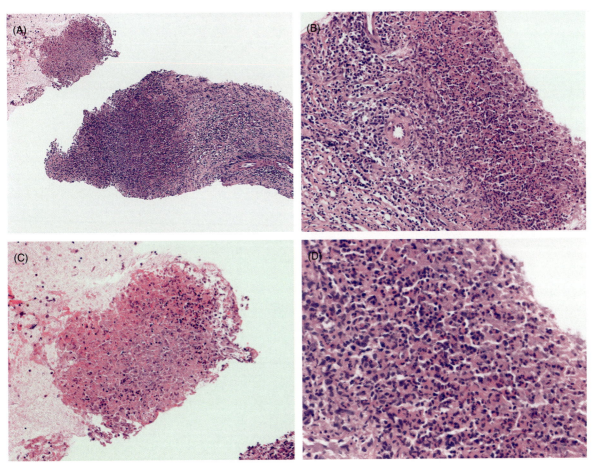

Illustrative case 2 (A–D) H&E sections show no identifiable normal nodal architecture. Instead there are areas of sclerosis, necrotic inflammatory exudate and an acute inflammatory infiltrate containing neutrophils and histiocytes. At high power (E) a population of histiocytic cells with elongated nuclei is seen. Ziehl–Neelsen staining (F–H) reveals numerous acid-fast bacteria within the histiocytes.

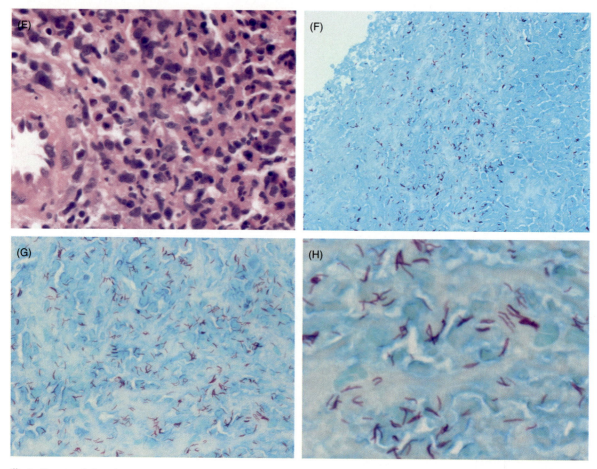

Illustrative case 2 (cont.)

Classical Hodgkin lymphoma

Classical Hodgkin lymphoma (CHL) is recognized in core biopsies by a loss of normal architecture, the presence of neoplastic cells with Hodgkin cell or Reed–Sternberg cell morphology (HRS cells), and a reactive background that contains a variable mixture of small lymphocytes, histiocytes, eosinophils, neutrophils, plasma cells and areas of fibrosis (Fig. 3.1A–D). The neoplastic HRS cells are large and may be mononuclear

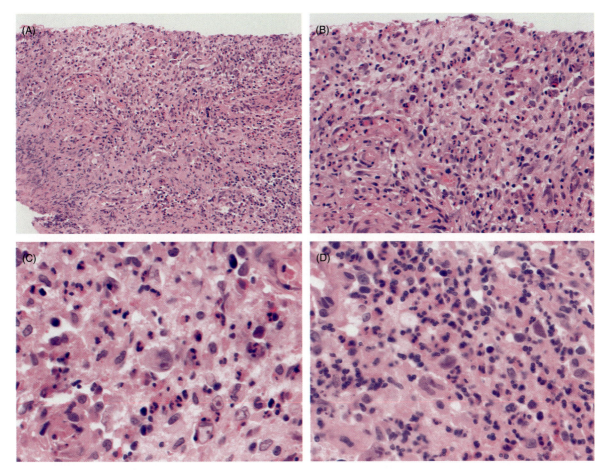

Figure 3.1 Classical Hodgkin lymphoma (CHL). (A–D) H&E sections from a core biopsy containing a sclerotic example of CHL. There is loss of the normal architecture with fibrosis and a mixed lymphoid infiltrate. Scattered large Hodgkin Reed–Sternberg (HRS) cells with multi-lobated nuclei and prominent nucleoli are seen on a background of histiocytes, neutrophils and eosinophils (C,D). Images (E) and (F) show a more cellular example of CHL. The architecture is effaced by a densely cellular infiltrate composed of small lymphocytes and larger HRS cells, some showing lacunar morphology (F). Image (G) is a high power view of a tumor cell-rich case of CHL that contains numerous lacunar cells and mummified cells with dense hyperchromatic nuclei. (H) CD30 staining of HRS, with membrane and Golgi positivity. CD15 can also show similar membrane and Golgi positivity (I). (J) PAX5 typically shows weak nuclear staining of HRS cells, which contrasts with the stronger positivity in background B cells. (K) CD20 can show focal positivity in HRS cells, and CD45 is typically negative (L).

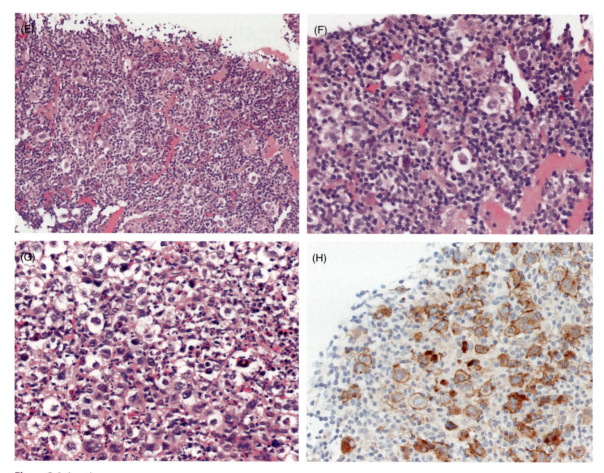

Figure 3.1 (cont.)

(Hodgkin cells) or multinucleated (Reed–Sternberg cells).[1] These HRS cells have abundant cytoplasm and contain large, often angular nuclei with frequent prominent eosinophilic nucleoli (Fig. 3.1C–G). Mummified forms with dense hyperchromatic nuclei and lacunar forms with clearing of the cytoplasm around the nucleus can also be seen (Fig. 3.1G).[2] The four histological subtypes of CHL – nodular sclerosis, mixed cellularity, lymphocyte-rich and lymphocyte-depleted – show differences in the reactive background and the morphology of the HRS cells. The nodular sclerosis subtype is usually the most readily identifiable, showing dense bands of collagenous fibrous tissue effacing the normal architecture and dividing up the residual lymphoid component into distinct nodules. Other subtypes may be less distinctive, and CHL cases can show a wide range of morphological variation – the disease may show an interfollicular pattern of distribution,[3] there can be numerous HRS cells grouped together to form

aggregates and sheets (the "syncytial variant"[4]), cases may show focal areas of necrosis, often surrounded by HRS cells, the background histiocytes can be numerous and may form granulomas, and background fibroblasts may predominate to give the appearance of a fibrous proliferation. With such a variable picture and the limited amount of material present in a needle core biopsy, it is not possible to assign a specific subtype to every case of CHL.

Although the recognition of the HRS cell is key to the diagnosis of CHL, the classical Reed–Sternberg cell with a bi-lobed nucleus and "owl's eye" nucleoli is rare in these specimens and may be completely absent in some biopsies. Whether this relates to tissue fixation effects or to traumatic artefact is not clear, but in needle biopsies many HRS cells lack specific identifiable features. They are seen as large atypical cells, some with eosinophilic nuclei, sometimes with lacunar cytoplasm and sometimes with a mummified appearance. Within

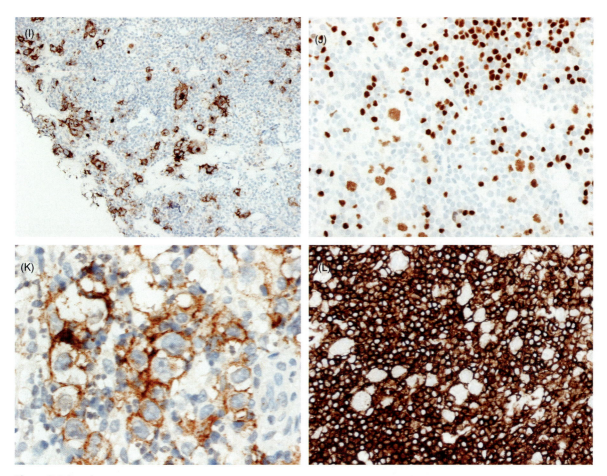

Figure 3.1 (cont.)

the biopsy the HRS cells are often grouped in loose clusters or nodules and, in contrast to the neoplastic cells in anaplastic large cell lymphoma, are rarely in contact with each other (the syncytial variant being the exception). The frequent lack of distinctive HRS morphology means that immunohistochemistry is often required to confirm the diagnosis of CHL.

The background in CHL needle core biopsies is also extremely variable.[5] Although there is usually stromal fibrosis in the nodular sclerosis subtype, the nodularity is not always apparent (Fig. 3.1A–D). Whilst eosinophils are a feature in many cases, some show a predominance of neutrophils (Fig. 3.1C,D) and others may lack both these cell types. In rare cases eosinophils or neutrophils can collect together to form microabscesses; these are often surrounded by HRS cells. The lymphocyte depleted subtype can be highly problematic. Cases with numerous histiocytes can be mistaken for a histiocytic neoplasm and cases with excessive fibroblasts may not be recognized as lymphoma.

Immunohistochemistry

The phenotype of the HRS cells is key to the diagnosis of CHL,[6] and the basic antibody panel includes CD30, CD15, PAX5, CD3, CD20, CD45 and EBER in-situ hybridization. CD30 positivity is an absolute requirement, and ideally should stain the cell membrane and show "dot-like" enhancement in the Golgi apparatus, although sometimes staining is cytoplasmic (Fig. 3.1H). In most cases CD30 positivity is strong; one should be wary of diagnosing CHL when there is only weak staining and an absence of CD30 positivity effectively excludes CHL. CD15 positivity in the large cells is helpful, but is not seen in all cases and may be very focal. Ideal staining resembles that of CD30 – membrane and Golgi (Fig. 3.1I) – but many cases show only patchy granular cytoplasmic positivity or are negative with this antibody. Remember that CD15 is not a specific marker – some histiocytes can express CD15 and it can be positive in T cell lymphomas. In the majority of CHL cases the

Table 3.1 Extended table of antibodies useful in the diagnosis of CHL

Antibody	Specificity	Utility
CD30	HRS cells, transformed lymphoid cells	Positivity required for the diagnosis of CHL
CD15	HRS cells (some cases), myeloid cells, macrophages	Positivity in HRS cells helpful, but negative in many cases and not specific
PAX5	B cell marker – protein regulator expressed in early stages of B cell differentiation	Weak nuclear positivity in HRS cells helpful. Positivity excludes ALCL; some cases very weak/negative
CD3	T cell marker – part of the protein complex associated with the T cell receptor	Stains background reactive T lymphocytes in most cases of CHL
CD20	Glycosylated phosphoprotein expressed on the surface of B cells	Negative or focal/heterogeneous staining of HRS cells
CD45	Leukocyte common antigen	HRS cells are negative; interpretation difficult
EBER ISH	EBV-encoded viral RNA	HRS cells positive in a percentage of CHL cases (EBV-LMP1 as alternative)
OCT-2	B cell transcription factor	Positive in most cases of DLBCL and in the LP cells of NLPHL. Stains 5–10% of CHL cases. Positivity with OCT-2 *and* BOB1 is not seen in HRS cells
BOB1	Lymphoctye transcription co-factor	Marks B cells in DLBCL and LP cells in NLPHL. Usually negative in HRS cells. Positivity with OCT-2 *and* BOB1 is not seen in HRS cells
CD10	Common ALL antigen positive in germinal center B cells	Negative in HRS cells. Positive in a subset of DLBCL
Bcl-6	Transcription factor expressed in the nuclei of germinal center B cells	There may be weak nuclear positivity in HRS cells. Strong nuclear staining is seen in the LP cells of NLPHL. Also positive in a subset of DLBCL cases
Bcl-2	Apoptosis regulator over-expressed in most cases of follicular lymphoma	Positive in HRS cells and in most other lymphomas. Not diagnostically helpful
MUM1/IRF4	B cell proliferation and differentiation marker	Positive in HRS cells and in subset of DLBCL. Negative in LP cells in NLPHL
ALK1	Anaplastic lymphoma kinase	Positive in ALCL, ALK positive. Negative in HRS cells
Cytotoxic markers	Granzyme B, Perforin and TIA1 – markers of cytotoxic T cells	Strong expression in ALCL. Negative/weakly positive in HRS cells
CD79a	B cell antigen receptor alpha chain	B cell marker; negative in the majority of HRS cells
CD19	B cell antigen	B cell marker; negative in the majority of HRS cells
CD22	B cell antigen	B cell marker; negative in the majority of HRS cells
Light chains	Immunoglobulin light chains produced by effective B cells	Light chain restriction is not seen in HRS cells, which are unable to produce antibody

Abbreviations: ALCL, anaplastic large cell lymphoma; ALL, acute lymphoblastic leukemia; CHL, classical Hodgkin lymphoma; DLBCL, diffuse large B cell lymphoma; EBV, Epstein–Barr virus; LP, lymphocyte predominant; NLPHL, nodular lymphocyte predominant Hodgkin lymphoma.

HRS cells will show weak nuclear positivity with PAX5 (Fig. 3.1J).[7] Positivity with this B cell marker is helpful in the exclusion of anaplastic large cell lymphoma. The staining should be less strong than is seen in normal B cells; in some cases it is extremely weak and very occasionally can be completely negative. The background lymphocytes in most cases of CHL are T cells and will be CD3 positive; lymphocyte-rich CHL is the exception, but this subtype is hard to recognize in core biopsies. In rare cases the HRS cells can express CD3 or other T cell markers. In the majority of cases the HRS cells are CD20 negative but some cases show positive CD20 staining (Fig. 3.1K), although this is usually weak and/or heterogeneous. Strong uniform CD20 staining raises the suspicion of diffuse large B cell lymphoma or a "gray zone" lymphoma (see below). The use of alternative B cell markers such as CD79a and CD19 is helpful in such cases; positivity with either or both of these antibodies is extremely rare in HRS cells and would support an alternative diagnosis. HRS cells are negative with CD45 (Fig. 3.1L), but there are a large number of CD45-positive cells present in most CHL biopsies so that interpretation of this stain can be difficult. Epstein–Barr virus (EBV) positivity in HRS cells is very helpful, although not present in all cases.[8] EBER in-situ hybridization is the most sensitive technique, but EBV-LMP1 immunohistochemistry can also be used. Table 3.1 lists an extended panel of antibodies that may be required to identify CHL and to exclude other conditions in the differential diagnosis.

Differential diagnosis

Classical Hodgkin lymphoma has a broad differential diagnosis. The main problem areas involve a distinction from diffuse large B cell lymphoma (DLBCL), B cell lymphoma unclassifiable with features intermediate between DLBCL and CHL ("gray zone" lymphoma), nodular lymphocyte predominant Hodgkin lymphoma (NLPHL), anaplastic large cell lymphoma (ALCL) and reactive hyperplasia. This is a highly complex area, and difficult cases often require extensive immunohistochemical investigation (Table 3.1).

Classical Hodgkin lymphoma: problems and pitfalls of core biopsies

- Typical Reed–Sternberg cells are rare in core biopsies, and the Hodgkin cells often lack typical "textbook" morphology (Fig. 3.1G). In the absence of characteristic morphology, large cells need to have the correct phenotype and an appropriate background population should be present in order to confirm the diagnosis of CHL.
- Large cells with HRS morphology can be seen in reactive conditions, many of which contain CD30-positive large cells with prominent nucleoli. The paracortical changes in infectious mononucleosis or dermatopathic lymphadenopathy should not be mistaken for CHL. Transforming B immunoblasts in a reactive lymph node will also be CD30 positive, and are not HRS cells. Reactive B immunoblasts often show a

peri-follicular distribution, and will be IgM positive and show polytypic light chain staining.
- Interfollicular CHL can be particularly difficult to diagnose. The biopsy will often contain only a limited interfollicular component between the reactive lymphoid follicles. Unless there are definite HRS cells with the correct phenotype and an appropriate background it may be advisable to ask for a repeat biopsy.
- It may not be possible to recognize specific subtypes of CHL on a core biopsy. Sclerosis may not be nodular and representative background populations may be absent.

References

1. Foss HD, Marafioti T, Stein H. [Hodgkin lymphoma. Classification and pathogenesis]. *Pathologe* 2000;**21**:113–123.

2. Lorenzen J, Thiele J, Fischer R. The mummified Hodgkin cell: cell death in Hodgkin's disease. *J Pathol* 1997;**182**:288–298.

3. Doggett RS, Colby TV, Dorfman RF. Interfollicular Hodgkin's disease. *Am J Surg Pathol* 1983;**7**:145–149.

4. Strickler JG, Michie SA, Warnke RA, Dorfman RF. The "syncytial variant" of nodular sclerosing Hodgkin's disease. *Am J Surg Pathol* 1986;**10**:470–477.

5. Eberle FC, Mani H, Jaffe ES. Histopathology of Hodgkin's lymphoma. *Cancer J* 2009;**15**:129–137.

6. Chittal SM, Cavérivière P, Schwarting R, et al. Monoclonal antibodies in the diagnosis of Hodgkin's disease. The search for a rational panel. *Am J Surg Pathol* 1988;**12**:9–21.

7. Torlakovic E, Torlakovic G, Nguyen PL, Brunning RD, Delabie J. The value of anti-pax-5 immunostaining in routinely fixed and paraffin-embedded sections: a novel pan pre-B and B-cell marker. *Am J Surg Pathol* 2002;**26**:1343–1350.

8. Wu TC, Mann RB, Charache P, et al. Detection of EBV gene expression in Reed–Sternberg cells of Hodgkin's disease. *Int J Cancer* 1990;**46**:801–804.

Illustrative case: Classical Hodgkin lymphoma

Illustrative case

History: Female aged 50. Human immunodeficiency virus (HIV)-positive patient, presenting with neck, chest and abdominal lymphadenopathy.

Comments: The core biopsy shows complete loss of the normal architecture, with a fibrous stromal background and a mixed cellular infiltrate containing small lymphocytes, histiocytes and numerous large atypical cells. The large cells show hyperchromatic and atypical nuclei and a high degree of pleomorphism. A few scattered cells show typical Reed–Sternberg morphology. Many cells show cytoplasmic clearing. The large cells show the phenotype of classical Hodgkin lymphoma. CD30 is positive, staining the cytoplasmic membranes and the Golgi apparatus. A few of the HRS cells are CD15 positive, showing typical granular cytoplasmic staining. The same cells show weak nuclear positivity with PAX5; the staining contrasts with the strong nuclear positivity in the background reactive B cells. The HRS are positive with EBER in-situ hybridization and are negative for CD3 and CD20.

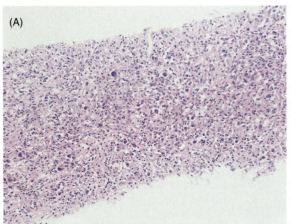
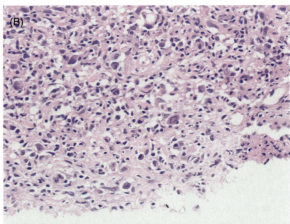

Illustrative case (A–C) H&E stains from a core biopsy in which there is effacement of the architecture by a mixed infiltrate containing prominent large atypical cells. The large cells (C) show hyperchromatic nuclei and prominent nucleoli with some bi-nucleate forms. CD30 staining is shown in (D); note the dot-like Golgi positivity in some cells. Focal granular cytoplasmic CD15 positivity is seen in occasional Hodgkin or Reed–Sternberg (HRS) cells (E). Image (F) shows the typical weak nuclear positivity with PAX5; background B cells show strong nuclear staining. The HRS cells in this case are Epstein–Barr virus (EBV)-positive; nuclear EBER staining is shown in (G). The background lymphocytes are mainly CD3-positive T cells (H). CD20 (I) shows only rare B cells; the HRS cells are negative.

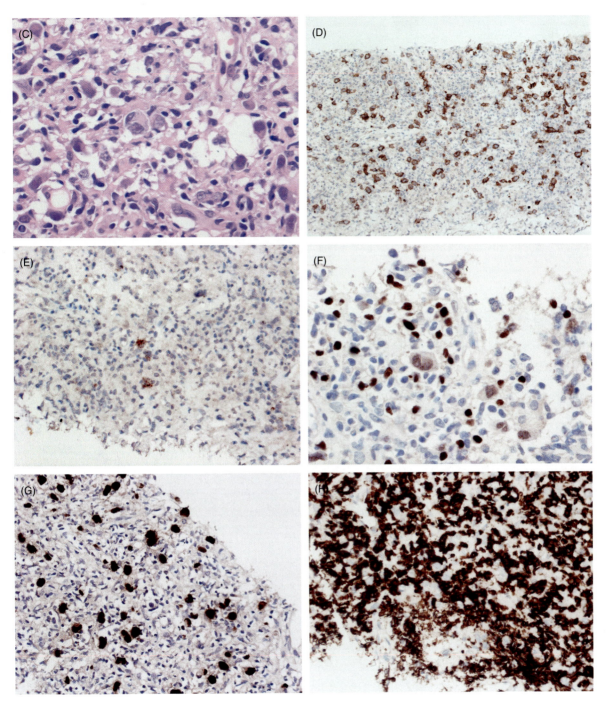

Illustrative case (cont.)

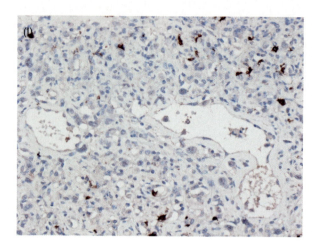

Illustrative case (cont.)

Classical Hodgkin lymphoma is a known human immunodeficiency virus (HIV)-related lymphoma, and most cases are EBV positive. The HRS cells in this case show a marked degree of nuclear pleomorphism, and typical Reed–Sternberg cells are very rare. The value of PAX5 staining is that it confirms the B cell nature of the neoplastic cells, and effectively excludes anaplastic large cell carcinoma, which should be in the differential diagnosis on morphology. In some cases the HRS cells can show focal or heterogeneous positivity with CD20. Nucleolar staining with CD20 (as seen faintly here) is non-specific. As in many core biopsies, it is difficult to identify the specific subtype of classical Hodgkin lymphoma in this case, but the large number of neoplastic cells and paucity of background lymphocytes suggest the lymphocyte-depleted variant.

Nodular lymphocyte predominant Hodgkin lymphoma

Nodular lymphocyte predominant Hodgkin lymphoma (NLPHL) is characterized by replacement of the normal nodal architecture with nodules composed of small lymphocytes, histiocytes and large cells known as LP (lymphocyte predominant) cells (Fig. 4.1A–E).[1,2] The large cells, previously called L&H cells (lymphocytic and histiocytic variant of Reed–Sternberg cells), are present within and just outside the nodules and show variable morphological features.[3] Many have a nucleus with a convoluted or folded outline said to resemble a kernel of popcorn – the "popcorn" cells. Other LP cells resemble large centroblasts or immunoblasts. The nuclei are generally pale and contain single or multiple nucleoli that are smaller and less eosinophilic than those of HRS cells. There is usually a moderate amount of cytoplasm, but some examples have abundant clear cytoplasm reminiscent of the lacunar cells in classical Hodgkin lymphoma (CHL) (Fig. 4.1D). Some "mummified" nuclei may also be present (Fig. 4.1D). In most cases of NLPHL it is possible to find LP cells with prominent eosinophilic nuclei that on an individual basis are indistinguishable from typical Reed–Sternberg cells (Fig. 4.1E). The background population consists of small mature lymphocytes and pale histiocytes, the latter often clustered together to form loose granulomas. Eosinophils, neutrophils and plasma cells are usually lacking, and most cases of NLPHL do not show significant sclerosis, although this can be a feature in chronic and/or recurrent disease.

The LP cells show a characteristic immunophenotype that is distinct from that of HRS cells in CHL.[4] There is expression of all B lineage markers – CD20, CD79a, PAX5 (strong nuclear positivity, in contrast with HRS cells), CD19 and CD22 (Fig. 4.1F, G) – and T cell markers are negative (Fig. 4.1H). There is a partial germinal center cell phenotype; the LP cells are CD10 negative, bcl-6 positive, OCT-2 strongly positive and BOB1 positive (Fig. 4.1I–K).[5,6] Bcl-2 is often negative but can be positive in some cases. The LP cells are able to produce immunoglobulin, and can show light chain restriction (Fig. 4.1L,M)[3] and expression of heavy chains, often IgD.[7] EMA is positive in approximately 50% of cases (Fig. 4.1N) and most cases are CD30 and CD15 negative (Fig. 4.1O,P), although some LP cells can express CD30. EBER is negative and MIB1 or Ki67 show that the majority of the LP cells are in cycle. The nodules show an underlying meshwork of follicular dendritic cells (FDCs) which can be demonstrated by CD21 staining (Fig. 4.1Q).[7] The small lymphocytes within the nodule are predominantly B cells (Fig. 4.1F), and are a mixture of mantle zone cells (IgM positive, IgD positive and bcl-2 positive) and some residual germinal center cells (CD10 positive, bcl-6 positive, bcl-2 negative). The nodules also contain an admixed T cell population, and T cells are frequently seen to ring the LP cells forming distinct "rosettes" (Fig. 4.1H). These rosetting T cells show a T follicular helper phenotype and are CD3 positive, CD4 positive, CD57 positive and PD1 positive (Fig. 4.1R).[8] The histiocytes will stain with CD68 and CD11c.

Differential diagnosis

1. Classical Hodgkin lymphoma.[9] The distinction between CHL and NLPHL is critical for the patient, and can be problematic in a core biopsy. The morphological overlap between LP cells and HRS cells means that it is not always possible to distinguish the two cell types on routine H&E sections. Key findings in NLPHL are an absence of CD30 and CD15 staining, well-defined positivity with B lineage markers (CD79a is particularly useful here, as it is negative in the HRS cells in almost all cases of CHL) and strong nuclear staining with OCT-2. Unlike HRS cells, LP cells may be EMA positive and light chain restriction, where present, effectively excludes CHL. The presence of CD21-positive FDC networks is also extremely helpful, although these can also be seen in the lymphocyte-rich subtype of CHL.[10]

2. Follicular lymphoma (FL). The nodular architecture, presence of FDC networks and

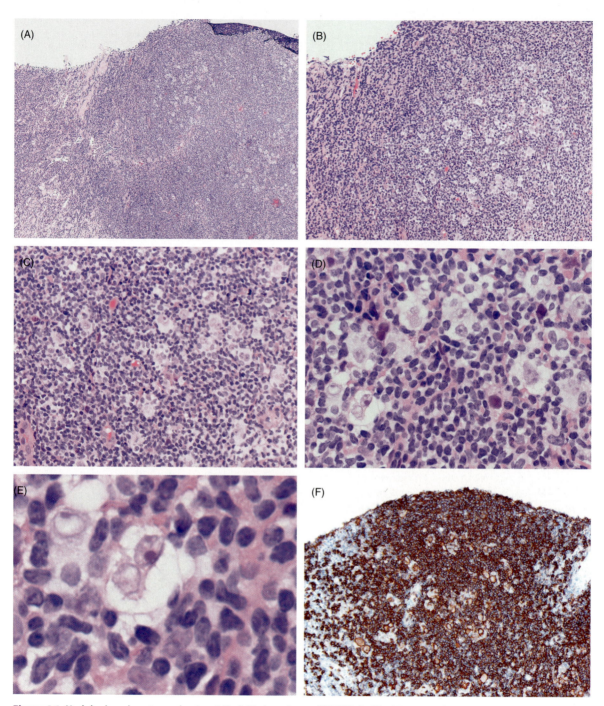

Figure 4.1 Nodular lymphocyte predominant Hodgkin lymphoma (NLPHL). (A–D) H&E sections from NLPHL. At low power there is a loss of the normal architecture and a vaguely nodular lymphoid infiltrate within which some large cells can be seen. At higher power the large cells are associated with pale histiocytes (D). The morphology of the large cells varies; some show a lacunar appearance, some are mummified (D), and occasional examples resemble Reed–Sternberg cells (E). Both the background lymphocytes and the LP cells are CD20 positive (F) and CD79a positive (G), with unstained T cells forming rosettes around the LP cells. CD3 shows a moderate number of background T lymphocytes and highlights the T cell rosettes around the LP cells (H). The LP cells are CD10 negative (I) and show strong nuclear expression of bcl-6 (J) and OCT-2 (K). In some cases the LP cells can show light chain restriction (kappa, L and lambda, M). EMA is expressed by the LP cells in a proportion of cases (N). CD30 and CD15 are usually negative on the LP cells (O,P). CD21 staining shows nodular follicular dendritic cell networks that surround many of the LP cells (Q). The T cell rosettes around the LP cells can be highlighted with PD1 (R).

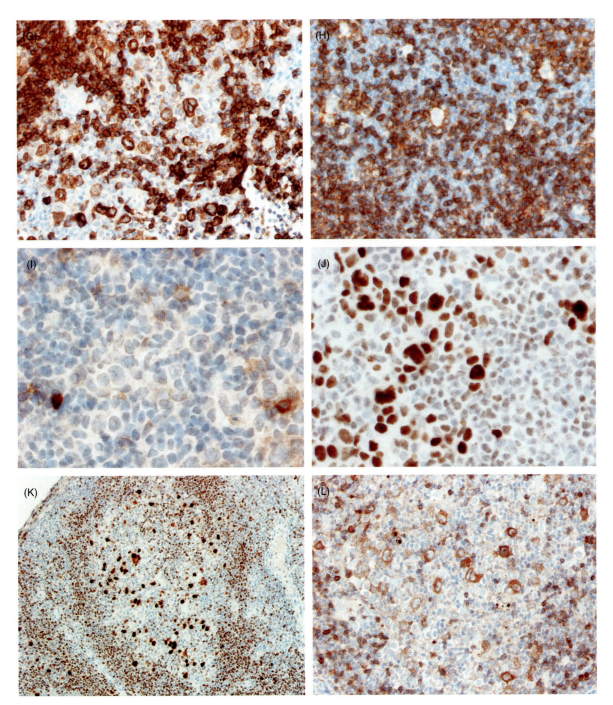

Figure 4.1 (cont.)

partial expression of germinal center cell markers can lead to NLPHL being mistakenly diagnosed as FL. In this setting the LP cells are incorrectly interpreted as centroblasts and the background lymphocytes as small centrocytes. Clues to the correct diagnosis include the presence of clusters of histiocytes (rare in FL), the recognition of LP cell morphology, the LP cell phenotype (CD10 negative, often bcl-2 negative, EMA positive), the rosetting of LP cells by T cells and the overall

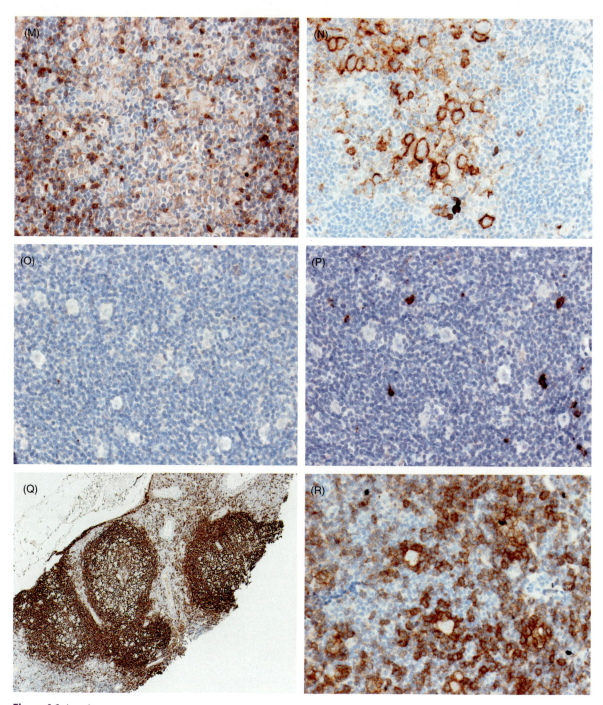

Figure 4.1 (cont.)

paucity of cells with a true germinal center cell phenotype.

3. T cell/histiocyte-rich large B cell lymphoma (THRLBCL).[11,12] These two conditions can show identical histology on core biopsies. Clinical information is critical here; NLPHL is usually localized disease whereas THRLBCL is frequently disseminated with hepatosplenomegaly and systemic symptoms. The neoplastic large B cells in THRLBCL and the LP cells of NLPHL can be

morphologically and phenotypically identical, and it may not always be possible to distinguish these two entities (see pitfalls below). Both may show the same partial expression of germinal center markers and both can be EMA positive. However the identification of well-defined FDC networks by definition excludes THRLBCL. The presence of a relatively large B cell population (mantle zone cells and residual germinal center cells) favors NLPHL, as does T cell rosetting and IgD expression by the large cells. In addition, the background T cells in THRLBCL are predominantly CD8 and cytotoxic marker positive, in contrast to the CD4-positive, CD57-positive, PD1-positive T cells in NLPHL.

4. Progressive transformation of germinal centers (PTGC).[13] This reactive condition is very difficult to diagnose in core biopsy, where only a small sample of the node is seen. The transformed follicles in PTGC contain residual clusters of germinal center cells separated by mantle zone lymphocytes. The larger germinal center cells may resemble LP cells. Helpful findings are positive staining with CD10 in the large germinal center cells, identifiable groups of germinal center cells (CD10 positive, bcl-6 positive, bcl-2 negative with a high MIB1 proliferation fraction) in the transformed follicle and a lack of T cell rosettes. The presence of residual normal reactive germinal centers in the biopsy may also be useful – it is rare to see these in NLPHL.

Nodular lymphocyte predominant Hodgkin lymphoma: problems and pitfalls of core biopsies

- Cases with few FDCs (sampling error) or diffuse forms of NLPHL are very difficult to diagnose and may need further biopsies.
- CD30 can stain up bystander (background) immunoblasts as well as the LP cells in some cases of NLPHL. The finding of CD30 positivity should not of itself lead to a diagnosis of CHL.
- Do not over-interpret EMA staining. This antibody is relatively non-specific and will stain up background histiocytes and plasma cells. Ensure that positive cells show LP cell morphology.
- Although typically nodular with a predominant population of small B cells in the background, there are cases of NLPHL with a more diffuse

architecture and with numerous T cells. In general the more chronic cases show more T cells, and provided the other features are present it should still be possible to make a diagnosis of NLPHL. A "nodular with T cell rich background" pattern has been described.[14] Where the architecture is more diffuse the situation is much more difficult. Cases with a predominantly diffuse pattern may represent sampling error, in that only part of the biopsy contains well-defined nodules, may be examples of NLPHL with diffuse architecture ("T cell rich B cell lymphoma like") or may represent THRLBCL rather than NLPHL (see below).

- The problems of distinguishing NLPHL and THRLBCL are mentioned in the differential diagnosis section above. Even with a full phenotype and knowledge of the clinical features it is sometimes necessary to issue a guarded report along the lines of "appearances favor nodular lymphocyte predominant Hodgkin lymphoma, but T cell/histiocyte rich large B cell lymphoma cannot be fully excluded."

References

1. Mason DY, Banks PM, Chan J, et al. Nodular lymphocyte predominance Hodgkin's disease. A distinct clinicopathological entity. *Am J Surg Pathol* 1994;**18**:526–530.

2. Nogová L, Rudiger T, Engert A. Biology, clinical course and management of nodular lymphocyte-predominant Hodgkin lymphoma. *Hematology Am Soc Hematol Educ Program* 2006;**1**;266–72.

3. Schmid C, Sargent C, Isaacson PG. L and H cells of nodular lymphocyte predominant Hodgkin's disease show immunoglobulin light-chain restriction. *Am J Pathol* 1991;**139**:1281–1289.

4. von Wasielewski R, Werner M, Fischer R, et al. Lymphocyte-predominant Hodgkin's disease. An immunohistochemical analysis of 208 reviewed Hodgkin's disease cases from the German Hodgkin Study Group. *Am J Pathol* 1997;**150**:793–803.

5. Uherova P, Valdez R, Ross CW, Schnitzer B, Finn WG. Nodular lymphocyte predominant Hodgkin lymphoma. An immunophenotypic reappraisal based on a single-institution experience. *Am J Clin Pathol* 2003;**119**:192–198.

6. Browne P, Petrosyan K, Hernandez A, Chan JA. The B-cell transcription factors BSAP, OCT-2, and BOB.1 and the pan-B-cell markers CD20, CD22, and CD79a are useful in the differential diagnosis of classic Hodgkin lymphoma. *Am J Clin Pathol* 2003;**120**:767–777.

7. Prakash S, Fountaine T, Raffeld M, Jaffe ES, Pittaluga S. IgD positive L&H cells identify a unique subset of nodular lymphocyte predominant Hodgkin lymphoma. *Am J Surg Pathol* 2006;**30**:585–592.

8. Nam-Cha SH, Roncador G, Sanchez-Verde L, et al. PD-1, a follicular T-cell marker useful for recognizing nodular lymphocyte-predominant Hodgkin lymphoma. *Am J Surg Pathol* 2008;**32**:1252–1257.

9. Bräuninger A, Wacker HH, Rajewsky K, Küppers R, Hansmann ML. Typing the histogenetic origin of the tumor cells of lymphocyte-rich classical Hodgkin's lymphoma in relation to tumor cells of classical and lymphocyte-predominance Hodgkin's lymphoma. *Cancer Res* 2003;**63**:1644–1651.

10. Anagnostopoulos I, Hansmann ML, Franssila K, et al. European Task Force on Lymphoma project on lymphocyte predominance Hodgkin disease: histologic and immunohistologic analysis of submitted cases reveals two types of Hodgkin disease with a nodular growth pattern and abundant lymphocytes. *Blood* 2000;**96**:1889–1899.

11. Rüdiger T, Gascoyne RD, Jaffe ES, et al. Workshop on the relationship between nodular lymphocyte predominant Hodgkin's lymphoma and T cell/histiocyte-rich B cell lymphoma. *Ann Oncol* 2002;**13** Suppl 1: 44–51.

12. Boudová L, Torlakovic E, Delabie J, et al. Nodular lymphocyte-predominant Hodgkin lymphoma with nodules resembling T-cell/histiocyte-rich B-cell lymphoma: differential diagnosis between nodular lymphocyte-predominant Hodgkin lymphoma and T-cell/histiocyte-rich B-cell lymphoma. *Blood* 2003;**102**:3753–3758.

13. Smith LB. Nodular lymphocyte predominant Hodgkin lymphoma: diagnostic pearls and pitfalls. *Arch Pathol Lab Med* 2010;**134**:1434–1439.

14. Fan Z, Natkunam Y, Bair E, Tibshirani R, Warnke RA. Characterization of variant patterns of nodular lymphocyte predominant Hodgkin lymphoma with immunohistologic and clinical correlation. *Am J Surg Pathol* 2003;**27**:1346–1356.

4 Illustrative case: Nodular lymphocyte predominant Hodgkin lymphoma

Illustrative case

History: Female aged 57. Clusters of large lymph nodes in the left axillary tail of breast, suspicious for lymphoma.

Comments: The core biopsy is not particularly well preserved, so the morphology is not ideal. The H&E shows a loss of the normal architecture with an infiltrate composed of scattered large cells on a background of small cells. Nodularity is not obvious on the H&E sections and the morphology of the large cells is not distinctive. Both classical Hodgkin lymphoma and NLPHL would be considered, but the immunophenotypic features support the latter diagnosis.

Although the H&E does not look nodular, CD21 reveals FDC networks that are seen to surround the large cells. The large cells are CD20 positive, CD79a positive, CD10 negative, bcl-6 positive and OCT-2 positive.

This case shows some of the difficulties in recognizing NLPHL. There are some CD30-positive cells present, but these represent bystander immunoblasts rather than LP cells. CD15 staining is negative, as is EBER. This is an example of a case of NLPHL that has a prominent background T cell population, but the phenotype of the LP cells is typical, and PD1 shows that the T cells form distinct rosettes around the LP cells.

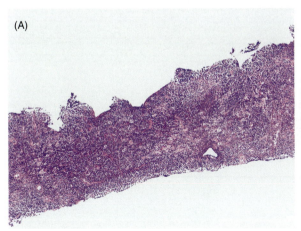
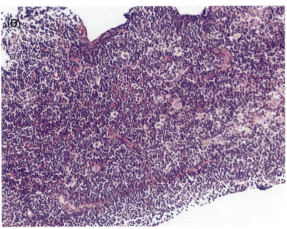

Illustrative case (A–E) H&E sections of the core biopsy from a case of nodular lymphocyte predominant Hodgkin lymphoma (NLPHL). At low power (A–C) there is effacement of the normal architecture by an apparently diffuse sheet of small lymphocytes which contains histiocytes and scattered larger cells. Images (D) and (E) show higher power pictures of the larger LP cells. The background small lymphocytes and the LP cells are positive for B cell markers (F is CD20 and G is CD79a). Note that the LP cells show negative "rosettes" of T cells. CD3 shows a significant T cell content in this case (H). CD21 staining reveals nodular networks of follicular dendritic cells (FDCs) that surround the LP cells (I). The LP cells are bcl-6 positive (J) and show strong nuclear positivity with OCT-2 (K). CD30 stains scattered "bystander" cells; the LP cells are negative (L) and CD15 is also negative (M). PD1 staining (N) highlights the T cell rosettes around the LP cells.

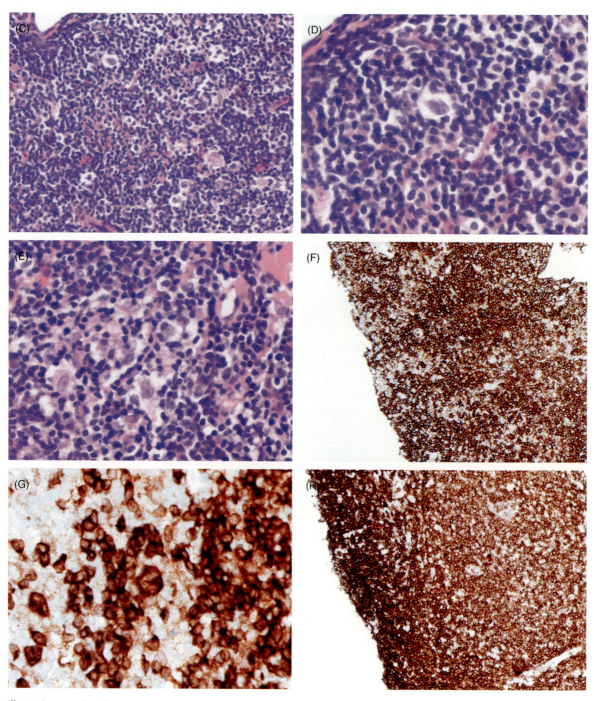

Illustrative case (cont.)

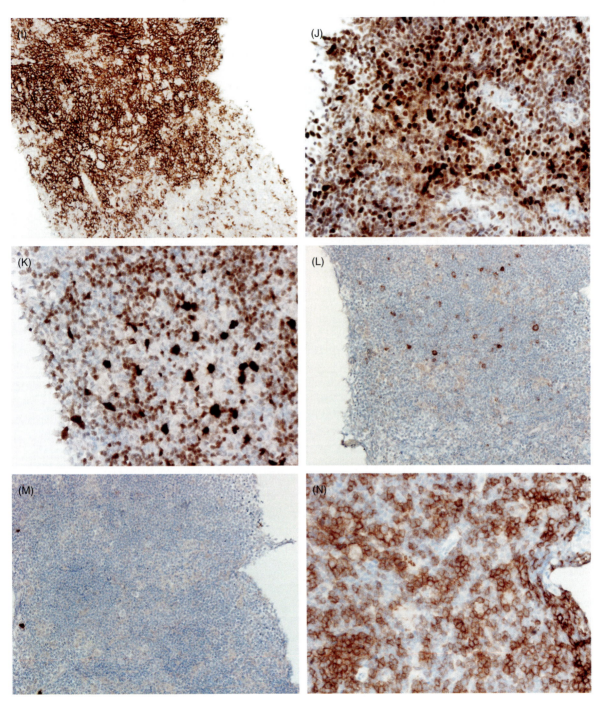

Illustrative case (cont.)

Chapter 5

Follicular lymphoma

Although a diagnosis of follicular lymphoma (FL) is frequently straightforward in excision specimens, it is often harder to recognize in needle core biopsies. The diagnosis is based on the identification of a follicular architecture and a population of cells with germinal center morphology and phenotype. The neoplastic follicles typically are uniform in size, lack tingible body macrophages and have poorly formed or absent mantle zones. They are made up of a mixture of centrocytes and centroblasts, with the numbers of the latter determining the grade of the tumor (Fig. 5.1A–E). Normal germinal center cells express B lineage markers (CD20, CD79a, PAX5; Fig. 5.1F),[1] are negative for T lineage markers (Fig. 5.1G) and are strongly positive with CD10 and bcl-6 (Fig. 5.1H,I).[2] In normal and reactive germinal centers the cells are bcl-2 negative, whereas in most FLs the neoplastic germinal center cells are bcl-2 positive (Fig. 5.1J).[3] CD21 stains the underlying follicular dendritic cells (FDCs), confirming a follicular architecture (Fig. 5.1K).[4] MIB1/Ki67 will usually show a low proliferation fraction, with no evidence of the zoned pattern seen in reactive germinal centers (Fig. 5.1L).[5] Light chain restriction can be helpful in identifying neoplastic germinal center cells[6] and in difficult cases fluorescence in-situ hybridization (FISH) can be used to look for the t(14;18) *bcl-2* translocation[7] and clonality can be demonstrated by polymerase chain reaction (PCR).[8]

Differential diagnosis

1. Reactive follicular hyperplasia. The changes seen in reactive lymph nodes are described in Chapter 1. Reactive germinal centers will normally have prominent tingible body macrophages and mantle zones, and the majority of the cells present will show centroblastic morphology. This contrasts with the monotonous population of centrocytes seen in the neoplastic follicles in the majority of

grade 1–2 FL cases. Bcl-2 staining is negative in reactive germinal centers and MIB1 is high and frequently shows zonation.[5]

2. Nodular lymphocyte predominant Hodgkin lymphoma (NLPHL). With nodules composed predominantly of small lymphocytes and underlying CD21-positive FDC networks, NLPHL can be mistaken for FL. The key is the identification of the LP cells (Chapter 4) and the absence of germinal center markers in the small B cells.

3. Extranodal marginal zone lymphoma (mucosa-associated lymphoid tissue (MALT) lymphoma) and FL can sometimes be difficult to distinguish. MALT lymphoma frequently contains reactive germinal centers, and the centrocyte-like tumor cells can resemble the centrocytes of FL. Identification of the reactive nature of the germinal centers (bcl-2 negative, high proliferation fraction) is important, as is the absence of germinal center cell markers in the centrocyte-like population (although bcl-6 can be weakly positive in MALT lymphoma). The finding of monocytoid or plasmacytic differentiation favors MALT lymphoma, and lymphoepithelial lesions (LELs) will be seen at some sites (salivary gland and thyroid in particular).[9]

4. Mantle cell lymphoma (MCL). The cells of MCL morphologically resemble centrocytes, and there can be a nodular or mantle zone pattern suggestive of a follicular architecture. In general the cells of MCL are more monomorphic than the mixed centrocytes and centroblasts in FL. CD21 can be misleading, as nodular MCL can be based around underlying follicles.

   Immunohistochemistry is critical, as the cells of MCL are CD5 and cyclin D1 positive. CD10 is negative in MCL, but there is often weak expression of bcl-6.

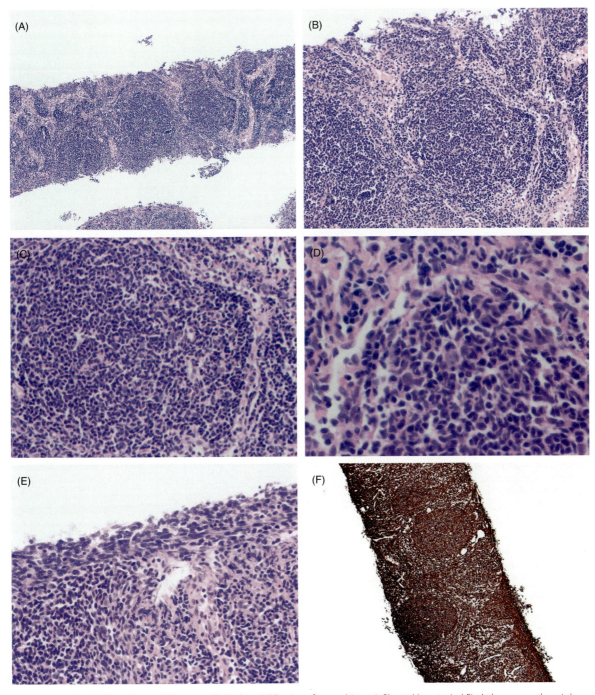

Figure 5.1 Follicular lymphoma (FL). Images (A–E) show H&E stains of a core biopsy infiltrated by a typical FL. At low power there is loss of the normal architecture and a follicular infiltrate. Occasional residual lymphoid sinuses are present between the follicles (A,B). The abnormal follicles lack tingible body macrophages and mantle zones and are composed predominantly of centrocytes, with very few nucleolated centroblasts (B–D). Image (E) shows a neoplastic follicle with the "streaming" effect at the edge of the biopsy. CD20 staining is shown in (F); note the presence of B cells in the interfollicular region. CD3 (G) shows T cells between the follicles and some intrafollicular T cells within the germinal centers. The germinal center cells, including those streaming at the edge of the biopsy are positive for CD10 (H) and bcl-6 (I). Bcl-2 is strongly expressed in the germinal centers (J) and CD21 (K) shows well-defined networks of follicular dendritic cells associated with the neoplastic follicles. MIB1 shows a low proliferation fraction within the neoplastic follicles (L).

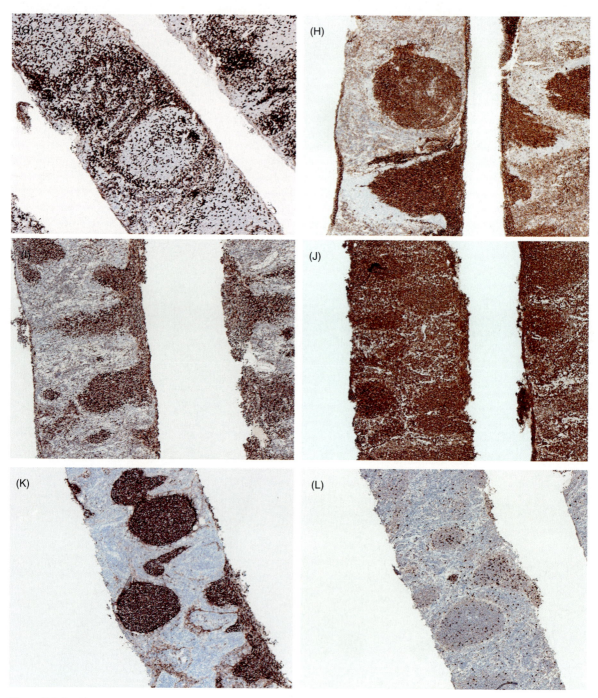

Figure 5.1 (cont.)

5. Chronic lymphocytic leukemia/small lymphocytic lymphoma (CLL/SLL). Nodes involved by CLL/SLL can show a nodular pattern that mimics FL at low power. Higher power shows a monomorphic population of mature small lymphocytes with proliferation centers rather than true follicles. The latter contain typical paraimmunoblasts. Immunohistochemistry shows

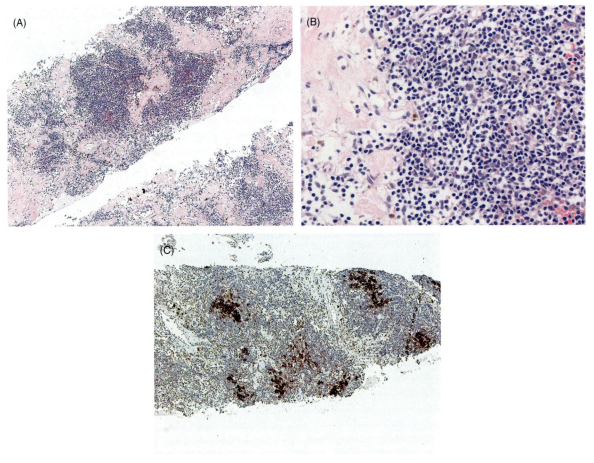

Figure 5.2 **Sclerotic follicular lymphoma (FL).** Sections illustrating a sclerotic case of FL from a retroperitoneal biopsy. On low power H&E (A) the lymphoid infiltrate lacks a follicular structure. At high power (B) both centroblasts and centrocytes can be identified. CD21 staining (C) reveals poorly defined follicular dendritic cell (FDC) networks and confirms a follicular architecture.

that the tumor cells are CD5 positive, CD23 positive, CD10 negative and bcl-6 negative. It should be noted that CD23 is not specific of itself – in some cases of FL the tumor cells are CD23 positive. Additionally, some CLL/SLL cases show weak expression of bcl-6. The proliferation centers in CLL/SLL can be highlighted with MIB1 or with MUM1, which stains paraimmunoblasts. CD21 may show some disrupted FDC networks but does not show an underlying follicular architecture.

Follicular lymphoma: problems and pitfalls of core biopsies

- Identification of a follicular architecture can be extremely difficult in core biopsies,

even using CD21. Where there is excessive sclerosis FDC networks are often minimal or even completely absent (Fig. 5.2A–C). This seems to be more frequent in biopsies from extranodal sites, particularly the bowel mesentery, peritoneum and retroperitoneum. In this setting expression of CD10 and bcl-6 are necessary for the diagnosis, and FISH studies may be helpful. In biopsies from these sites it is difficult or impossible to assign a specific World Health Organization pattern (follicular, follicular and diffuse, focally follicular or diffuse) to the lesion.

- The "pipestem" or "streaming" distortion of germinal centers described in reactive lymph nodes (see Chapter 1) is very common in

FL. Many of the neoplastic germinal centers are stretched out along the edges of the biopsy and occasionally this can make identification of follicles difficult. The nature of "streamed" germinal centers can be confirmed with CD10, bcl-6 and CD21 (Fig. 5.1E,H,I,K).

- The morphological features that distinguish reactive from neoplastic follicles are not absolute, and may lead to confusion in core biopsies where only a limited amount of tumor is available for assessment. The neoplastic follicles in FL can contain occasional tingible body macrophages, and some cases show relatively well-preserved mantle zones. The neoplastic follicles may show irregular outlines, and higher grade FL can contain frequent centroblasts (see below). In difficult cases, bcl-2 staining, light chain restriction and PCR are all useful.

- There are a large number of morphological variants of FL that can lead to diagnostic confusion. These include FL with monocytoid or marginal zone differentiation, FL with plasmacytic differentiation, "inverted" FL, "floral" FL and signet ring FL.[10–13] All of these may make FL hard to recognize in a core biopsy – germinal center cell markers should be included in the antibody panel for all small B cell lymphomas.

- There is a variable interfollicular component in FL – the neoplastic cells are not confined to the follicles. These interfollicular cells often downregulate germinal center cell markers and are frequently CD10 negative and bcl-6 weakly positive. Distinguishing an extensive interfollicular component from FL with a partial diffuse architecture (follicular and diffuse FL) can be problematic.

- There are pitfalls associated with bcl-2 staining. Firstly, expression of this antibody is variable and some cases are only weakly positive. Secondly, the existence of bcl-2 negative FL is well recognized.[14] In some examples the negativity is related to variations in the bcl-2 molecule leading to a loss of the epitope recognized by the commonest bcl-2 antibody, and use of alternative bcl-2 antibodies can lead to positive staining. In other bcl-2 negative FL cases the tumor cells appear to carry an alternative (*bcl-6*) translocation and do not show over-expression of bcl-2. It is also important not to over-interpret bcl-2 staining. Some reactive germinal centers will contain a high number of interfollicular T cells, which will express bcl-2. These should not be mistaken for neoplastic follicles.

- FL can show other phenotypic abnormalities, as well as those involving bcl-2. A subset of cases are CD10 negative, which can make recognition difficult.[15] Whilst MIB1 is usually low in FL, some cases show a high proliferation fraction yet retain low-grade cytological features. Some FL cases show a high percentage of T cells within the follicles, occasionally making it difficult to distinguish FL from the follicular variant of peripheral T cell lymphoma, not otherwise specified. PCR studies may be required to determine the tumor lineage.

- One particular area where needle core biopsies can present problems involves the distinction between grade 3 FL and diffuse large B cell lymphoma (DLBCL). Where there is a high centroblast content and where the follicular architecture is only partial or indistinct, it may not be possible to separate FL grade 3A from FL grade 3B or DLBCL. This is often the case when there is transformation of the FL into DLBCL. Since the presence of transformation to DLBCL has important implications for patient treatment, where the pathology findings are doubtful then a repeat (possibly excision) biopsy should be recommended.

- The potential difficulties in distinguishing FL from MALT lymphoma have been alluded to. It should be noted that although LELs are taken as a marker of MALT lymphoma, these can be found in cases of FL involving MALT sites (Fig. 5.3A–D).[9]

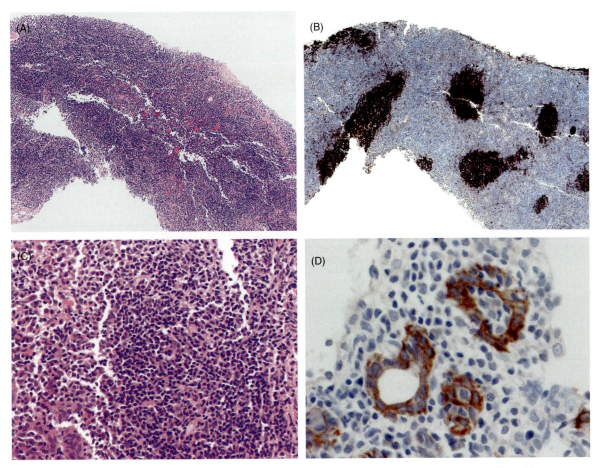

Figure 5.3 Follicular lymphoma (FL) of the thyroid. (A) A low power H&E from a core biopsy of a thyroid gland infiltrated by FL. Residual glandular tissue can be seen and the follicular architecture is not well defined. CD21 (B) shows follicular dendritic cell (FDC) networks confirming a follicular infiltrate. (C) A high power H&E showing glandular tissue at the bottom left and a neoplastic follicle on the right. The follicle is composed of centrocytes and is poorly circumscribed. The centrocytes are seen to invade into the glandular tissue. (D) A high power cytokeratin stain (MNF116) showing nests of centrocytes lying within the thyroid epithelium. This appearance can mimic the lymphoepithelial lesions seen in mucosa-associated lymphoid tissue (MALT) lymphoma.

References

1. Torlakovic E, Torlakovic G, Nguyen PL, Brunning RD, Delabie J. The value of anti-pax-5 immunostaining in routinely fixed and paraffin-embedded sections: a novel pan pre-B and B-cell marker. *Am J Surg Pathol* 2002;**26**:1343–1350.

2. Dogan A, Bagdi E, Munson P, Isaacson PG. CD10 and BCL-6 expression in paraffin sections of normal lymphoid tissue and B-cell lymphomas. *Am J Surg Pathol* 2000;**24**:846–852.

3. Séité P, Hillion J, d'Agay MF, et al. BCL2 gene activation and protein expression in follicular lymphoma: a report on 64 cases. *Leukemia* 1993;**7**:410–417.

4. Petrasch S, Brittinger G, Wacker HH, Schmitz J, Kosco-Vilbois M. Follicular dendritic cells in non-Hodgkin's lymphomas. *Leuk Lymphoma* 1994;**15**:33–43.

5. Bryant RJ, Banks PM, O'Malley DP. Ki67 staining pattern as a diagnostic tool in the evaluation of lymphoproliferative disorders. *Histopathology* 2006;**48**:505–515.

6. Gelb AB, Rouse RV, Dorfman RF, Warnke RA. Detection of immunophenotypic abnormalities in paraffin-embedded B-lineage non-Hodgkin's lymphomas. *Am J Clin Pathol* 1994;**102**:825–834.

7. Vaandrager JW, Schuuring E, Raap T, et al. Interphase FISH detection of BCL2 rearrangement in follicular lymphoma using breakpoint-flanking probes. *Genes Chromosomes Cancer* 2000;**27**:85–94.

8. Chen YT, Whitney KD, Chen Y. Clonality analysis of B-cell lymphoma in fresh-frozen and paraffin-embedded tissues: the effects of variable polymerase chain reaction parameters. *Mod Pathol* 1994;**7**:429–434.

9. Bacon CM, Diss TC, Ye H, et al. Follicular lymphoma of the thyroid gland. *Am J Surg Pathol* 2009;**33**:22–34.

10. Schmid U, Cogliatti SB, Diss TC, Isaacson PG. Monocytoid/marginal zone B-cell differentiation in follicle centre cell lymphoma. *Histopathology* 1996;**29**:201–208.

11. Gradowski JF, Jaffe ES, Warnke RA, et al. Follicular lymphomas with plasmacytic differentiation include two subtypes. *Mod Pathol* 2010;**23**:71–79.

12. Kojima M, Yamanaka S, Yoshida T, et al. Histological variety of floral variant of follicular lymphoma. *APMIS* 2006;**114**:626–632.

13. Kim H, Dorfman RF, Rappaport H. Signet ring cell lymphoma. A rare morphologic and functional expression of nodular (follicular) lymphoma. *Am J Surg Pathol* 1978;**2**:119–132.

14. Schraders M, de Jong D, Kluin P, Groenen P, van Krieken H. Lack of Bcl-2 expression in follicular lymphoma may be caused by mutations in the BCL2 gene or by absence of the t(14;18) translocation. *J Pathol* 2005;**205**:329–335.

15. Marafioti T, Copie-Bergman C, Calaminici M, et al. Another look at follicular lymphoma: immunophenotypic and molecular analyses identify distinct follicular lymphoma subgroups. *Histopathology* 2013;**62**:860–875.

Illustrative cases: Follicular lymphoma

Illustrative case 1

History: Female aged 59. Enlarged abdominal lymph nodes. Biopsy of a mesenteric node.

Comments: This core biopsy shows a follicular infiltrate. The follicles are small, lack mantle zones and tingible body macrophages and are mainly composed of centrocytes with scattered centroblasts. The morphology is that of follicular lymphoma (FL), grade 1–2. However, whilst the cells in the follicles are CD20 positive and CD21 confirms a follicular architecture, CD10 shows only occasional positive cells in the germinal centers and bcl-2 is negative.

This is an example of a bcl-2 negative FL which also lacked expression of CD10. This phenotype is present in a subset of FL. The morphology is reassuring here, and CD21, bcl-6 and MIB1 stains are fully compatible with the diagnosis of FL. Fluorescence in-situ hybridization (FISH) was carried out on this case and identified a t(14;18) translocation, providing molecular confirmation of the diagnosis.

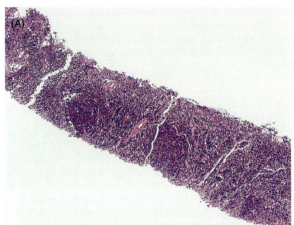
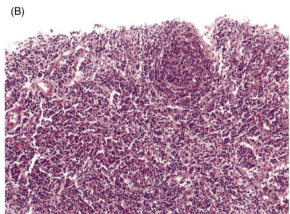

Illustrative case 1 (A–D) H&E sections from a core biopsy in which the normal architecture is effaced by a follicular infiltrate. The follicles are composed mainly of monomorphic centrocytes and show no mantle zones or tingible body macrophages. The infiltrate is CD20 positive (E) and CD3 (F) stains reactive T cells. CD21 confirms follicular dendritic cell networks associated with the follicles (G). CD10 staining (H) shows only a small number of positive cells within the follicles; in contrast bcl-6 (I) is positive in most of the cells in the follicle. Bcl-2 is negative in the germinal centers, but stains both interfolliclular and intrafollicular T cells (J). MIB1 (K) shows a low proliferation fraction in the neoplastic follicles, with no evidence of zonation.

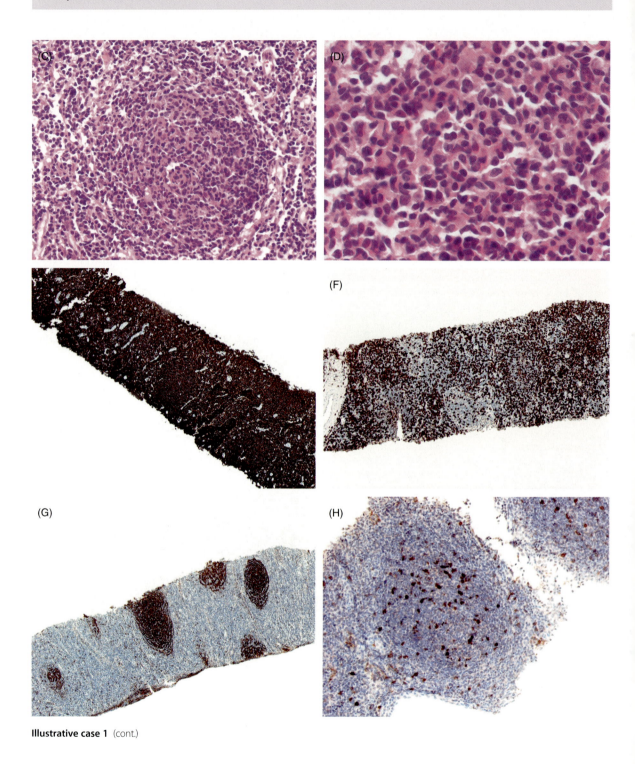

Illustrative case 1 (cont.)

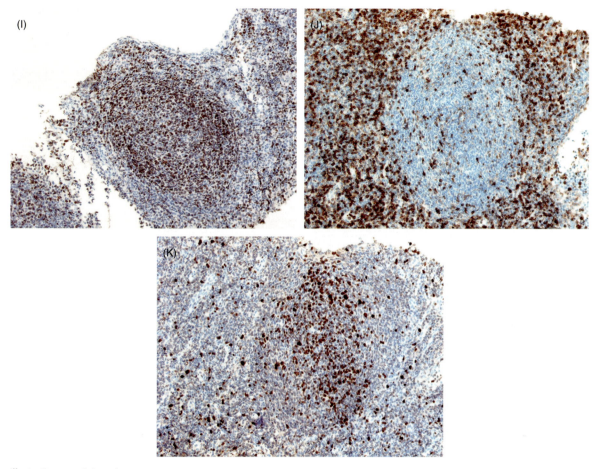

Illustrative case 1 (cont.)

Illustrative case 2

History: Female aged 62. History of diffuse large B cell lymphoma treated 18 months previously. Now enlarged right axillary node – possible relapse?

Comment: The H&E stains show a loss of the normal architecture and effacement by a vaguely nodular infiltrate. The infiltrate contains small cells with centrocyte morphology, a few centroblasts, and collections of cells with clear cytoplasmic vacuoles. These vacuoles compress the nucleus to the periphery of the cell leading to the signet ring morphology. Despite this unusual morphology, the infiltrating cells are CD20 positive, CD10 positive, bcl-6 positive and bcl-2 positive and CD21 shows an underlying follicular architecture. This is an example of a signet ring follicular lymphoma. The vacuoles in such cases are not mucin or immunoglobulin, and are probably due to accumulation of glycogen.

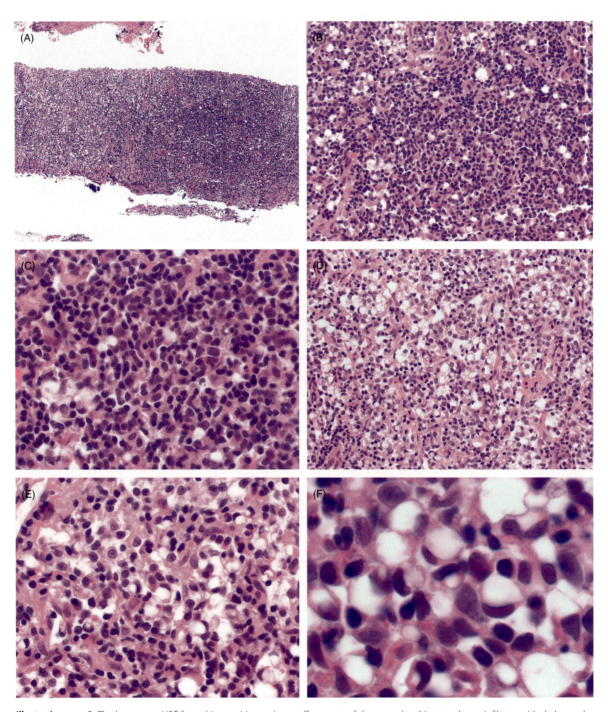

Illustrative case 2 The low power H&E from this core biopsy shows effacement of the normal architecture by an infiltrate with darker and lighter areas (A). The darker areas (B,C) show smaller cells with centrocytic morphology admixed with larger centroblastic cells. In the lighter areas (D–F) there are small and medium-sized lymphocytes and vacuolated cells with cytoplasmic clearing. Many of the latter show a "signet ring" appearance (F). The infiltrate (including the vacuolated cells) is CD20 positive (G) and CD10 positive (H). Bcl-6 staining is positive and shows some follicularity (I) and there is widespread bcl-2 positivity (J). CD21 (K) shows some distorted follicular dendritic cell networks indicating a partial follicular architecture.

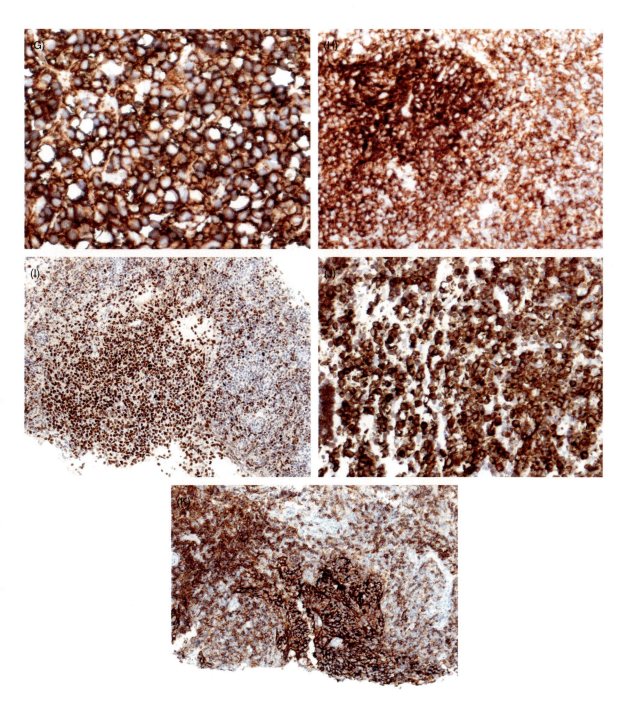

Illustrative case 2 (cont.)

Mantle cell lymphoma

Core biopsies from mantle cell lymphoma (MCL) normally show a monomorphic infiltrate of small to medium-sized cells with angular nuclei, absent or small nucleoli and minimal cytoplasm (Fig. 6.1A–D).[1,2] Occasionally there is a nodular pattern, and rarely the lesion is localized to the mantle zones, but these features are often difficult to discern in core biopsies. Hyalinized small blood vessels are often seen within the infiltrate, but are not a reliable diagnostic feature in core biopsies.

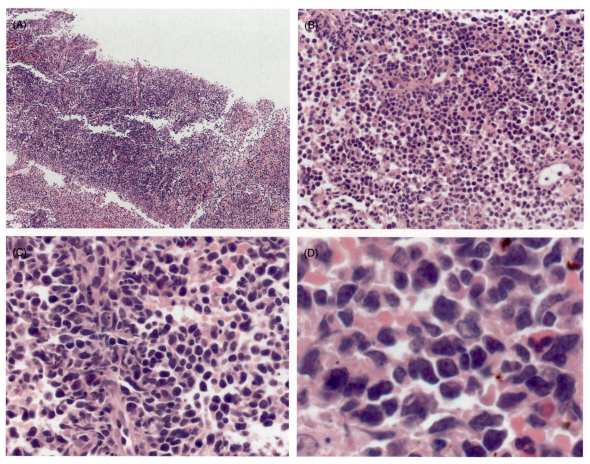

Figure 6.1 **Mantle cell lymphoma (MCL)**. Images (A–D) show the H&E appearances of MCL. At low power (A,B) the normal architecture is effaced by a rather ill-defined infiltrate composed of small lymphoid cells. In this example there are areas of oedema and the infiltrate is poorly cohesive. The tumor in this case is partly necrotic and the surviving cells show a perivascular pattern. At higher power (C,D) the tumor cell detail is visible. The cells are small to medium-sized with angulated dark nuclei and a small amount of eosinophilic cytoplasm. Nucleoli are small and multiple (D). The tumor cells are CD20 positive (E); CD79a was also positive (not illustrated). CD3 is negative (F) and CD5 is positive (G). Both cyclin D1 and SOX11 show nuclear positivity (H and I, respectively). Note the negative staining of the blood vessels and histiocytes with these antibodies. MIB1 (J) in this case shows a proliferation fraction of approximately 60%.

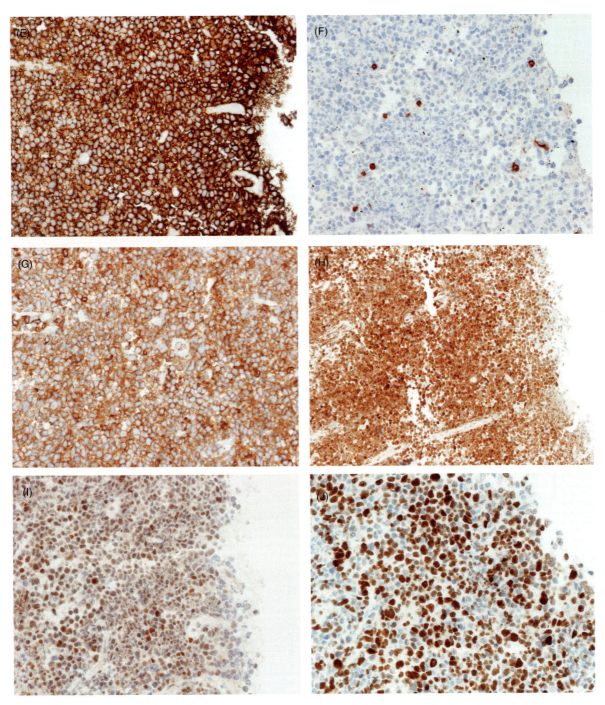

Figure 6.1 (cont.)

Scattered individual epithelioid histiocytes are often interspersed throughout the neoplastic lymphoid infiltrate. The tumor cells express B lineage markers as well as CD5 and cyclin D1 and SOX11 (Fig. 6.1E–I).[3] Bcl-2 is positive and germinal center markers are usually negative, although there can be weak positivity with bcl-6.[4] IgM and IgD are usually expressed and MUM1 is negative. MIB1 (Fig. 6.1J)

65

shows a variable proliferation fraction. The latter is of prognostic significance – patients where the tumor cell proliferation is over 30% are considered for more intensive therapy.[5] CD21 may show a loose background network of follicular dendritic cells (FDCs) in MCL.[6]

The pleomorphic and blastoid variants of MCL can be difficult to recognize. The cells in the pleomorphic variant are larger and show more prominent nucleoli, resembling a diffuse large B cell lymphoma (DLBCL). CD5 and cyclin D1 staining are required to confirm the diagnosis. The blastoid variant shows monomorphic featureless cells resembling lymphoblasts, and has a high mitotic rate and a proliferative index of over 60%.[7]

Differential diagnosis

1. MCL falls into a well-defined group of small B cell lymphomas – follicular lymphoma (FL), chronic lymphocytic leukemia/small lymphocytic lymphoma (CLL/SLL), marginal zone lymphoma (MZL) and lymphoplasmacytic lymphoma (LPL). Immunohistochemistry is frequently required to distinguish these entities, and this is summarized in Table 6.1.[8]

2. Other lymphomas that may mimic MCL include Burkitt lymphoma (BL) and B lymphoblastic leukemia/lymphoma. BL is recognized by the presence of prominent apoptoses, the expression of germinal center cell

Table 6.1 Extended table of antibodies used in the differential diagnosis of MCL and other small B cell lymphomas

Antibody	Specificity	Utility
CD20	Glycosylated phosphoprotein expressed on the surface of B cells	Confirms B lineage (may be negative in patients treated with rituximab)
CD79a	B cell antigen receptor alpha chain	Alternative B lineage marker (unaffected by rituximab)
PAX5	B cell marker – protein regulator expressed in early stages of B cell differentiation	Alternative B lineage marker (unaffected by rituximab) – nuclear stain
CD3	T cell marker – part of the protein complex associated with the T cell receptor	Stains background reactive T lymphocytes
CD5	T cell surface glycoprotein	Positive in B cells in MCL and in CLL/SLL
CD10	Common ALL antigen positive in germinal center B cells	Positive in FL (most cases); negative in MCL
Bcl-6	Transcription factor expressed in the nuclei of germinal center B cells	Positive in FL. May show weak nuclear positivity in MCL, CLL/SLL, MZL and LPL
Bcl-2	Apoptosis regulator over-expressed in most cases of FL	Positive in most cases of FL as well as in MCL, CLL/SLL, MZL and LPL
MUM1/IRF4	B cell proliferation and differentiation marker	Negative in MCL and most FL. Stains paraimmunoblasts in CLL/SLL and cells with plasmacytic differentiation in MZL and LPL
Cyclin D1	Cyclin protein involved in cell cycle regulation	Nuclear positivity in MCL. Negative in FL, CLL/SLL, MZL and LPL
SOX11	Transcription factor	Nuclear positivity in MCL. Negative in FL, CLL/SLL, MZL and LPL
CD23	B cell low affinity IgE receptor	Negative in MCL. Normally positive in CLL/SLL and positive in some cases of FL, MZL and LPL. Marks FDCs
CD138 (Syndecan)	Proteoglycan plasma cell marker	Positive in plasma cells in LPL and MZL. Negative in MCL, CLL/SLL and FL
TdT (Terminal deoxynucleotidyl transferase)	DNA polymerase expressed in immature lymphoid cells	Positive in B (and T)lymphoblastic leukemia/lymphoma
CD21	Complement receptor expressed on FDCs	Detects FDC networks in FL. MCL may show a loose background FDC network. Occasional tumor cell staining in FL, MZL and LPL
EBER	Epstein–Barr encoded viral RNA	Positive in a subset of Burkitt lymphoma. Negative in MCL

Abbreviations: ALL, acute lymphoblastic leukemia; CLL/SLL, chronic lymphocytic leukemia/small lymphocytic lymphoma; FDC, follicular dendritic cell; FL, follicular lymphoma; LPL, lymphoplasmacytic lymphoma; MCL, mantle cell lymphoma; MZL, marginal zone lymphoma.

markers, an absence of bcl-2 staining and a proliferation fraction of over 95% with MIB1. In addition some BL cases are Epstein–Barr virus (EBV) positive and will stain with EBER. Lymphoblastic leukemia/lymphoma is composed of monomorphic blast cells and can morphologically resemble MCL. Expression of TdT is helpful here, and many cases of B lymphoblastic leukemia/lymphoma will be CD10 and/or CD34 positive. MIB1 is usually high (over 60%) in most lymphoblastic lymphomas.

Mantle cell lymphoma: problems and pitfalls of core biopsies

- A percentage of MCL may be CD5 negative or only weakly positive. Cyclin D1 staining is necessary in all newly diagnosed small B cell lymphomas.[9]
- A percentage of MCL may be cyclin D1 negative;[10] usually CD5 positivity is retained. In some, but not all, cases SOX11 staining (Fig. 6.1I) will be positive.[11,12] Fluorescence in-situ hybridization (FISH) for the CCND1 translocation may be helpful.[13]
- Although bcl-6 is a marker of germinal center cells, weak positive staining is seen in a number of small B cell lymphomas, including MCL, MZL and CLL/SLL.
- The blastoid and pleomorphic variants of MCL can be problematic (see above). DLBCL frequently expresses germinal center cell markers (CD10, bcl-6, MUM1) and is typically negative with CD5 and cyclin D1, although CD5-positive cases and rare cyclin D1-positive cases are recorded.[14,15] Using FISH for the CCND1 translocation may be required in this setting.

References

1. Vandenberghe E. Mantle cell lymphoma. *Blood Rev* 1994;**8**:79–87.

2. Raffeld M, Sander CA, Yano T, Jaffe ES. Mantle cell lymphoma: an update. *Leuk Lymphoma* 1992;**8**:161–166.

3. Garcia-Conde J, Cabanillas F. Mantle cell lymphoma: a lymphoproliferative disorder associated with aberrant function of the cell cycle. *Leukemia* 1996;**10** Suppl 2: 78–83.

4. Gualco G, Weiss LM, Harrington WJ Jr, Bacchi CE. BCL6, MUM1, and CD10 expression in mantle cell lymphoma. *Appl Immunohistochem Mol Morphol* 2010;**18**:103–108.

5. Räty R, Franssila K, Joensuu H, Teerenhovi L, Elonen E. Ki-67 expression level, histological subtype, and the International Prognostic Index as outcome predictors in mantle cell lymphoma. *Eur J Haematol* 2002;**69**:11–20.

6. Manconi R, Poletti A, Volpe R, Sulfaro S, Carbone A. Dendritic reticulum cell pattern as a microenvironmental indicator for a distinct origin of lymphoma of follicular mantle cells. *Br J Haematol* 1988;**68**:213–218.

7. Ott G, Kalla J, Ott MM, et al. Blastoid variants of mantle cell lymphoma: frequent bcl-1 rearrangements at the major translocation cluster region and tetraploid chromosome clones. *Blood* 1997;**89**:1421–1429.

8. Chen CC, Raikow RB, Sonmez-Alpan E, Swerdlow SH. Classification of small B-cell lymphoid neoplasms using a paraffin section immunohistochemical panel. *Appl Immunohistochem Mol Morphol* 2000;**8**:1–11.

9. Bell ND, King JA, Kusyk C, Nelson BP, Sendelbach KM. CD5 negative diffuse mantle cell lymphoma with splenomegaly and bone marrow involvement. *South Med J* 1998;**91**:584–587.

10. Shiller SM, Zieske A, Holmes H 3rd, et al. CD5-positive, cyclin D1-negative mantle cell lymphoma with a translocation involving the CCND2 gene and the IGL locus. *Cancer Genet* 2011;**204**:162–164.

11. Xu W, Li JY. SOX11 expression in mantle cell lymphoma. *Leuk Lymphoma* 2010;**51**:1962–1967.

12. Zeng W, Fu K, Quintanilla-Fend L, et al. Cyclin D1-negative blastoid mantle cell lymphoma identified by SOX11 expression. *Am J Surg Pathol* 2012;**36**:214–219.

13. Li JY, Gaillard F, Moreau A, et al. Detection of translocation t(11;14)(q13;q32) in mantle cell lymphoma by fluorescence in situ hybridization. *Am J Pathol* 1999;**154**:1449–1452.

14. Yamaguchi M, Ohno T, Oka K, et al. De novo CD5-positive diffuse large B-cell lymphoma: clinical characteristics and therapeutic outcome. *Br J Haematol* 1999;**105**:1133–1139.

15. Rodriguez-Justo M, Huang Y, Ye H, et al. Cyclin D1-positive diffuse large B-cell lymphoma. *Histopathology* 2008;**52**:900–903.

Illustrative case: Mantle cell lymphoma

Illustrative case

History: Male aged 76. Presented with splenomegaly and disseminated lymphadenopathy. Biopsy of cervical lymph node (and bone marrow trephine biopsy).

Comments: The node shows a degree of background sclerosis and an infiltrate with the morphology of MCL. The typical phenotype is present – B lineage markers are positive together with CD5 and cyclin D1. Note that the cyclin D1 staining is heterogeneous, with some nuclei staining strongly and others showing only weak expression. As is often the case, bcl-6 also shows some nuclear staining, but this is much weaker than that seen in follicular lymphoma. A section from the bone marrow trephine showed deposits of MCL in the marrow, indicating (together with the splenomegaly) that the patient had Stage IV disease.

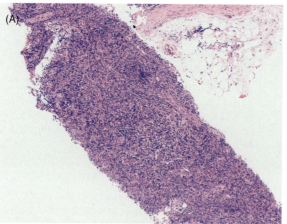
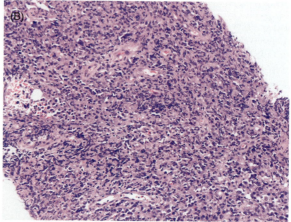

Illustrative case (A,B) Low power H&E sections from a core biopsy showing an effacement of the normal architecture by a monomorphic cellular infiltrate with a prominent vascular pattern. The tumor cells show angulated nuclei lacking in nucleoli (C,D) and are CD20 positive (E; note negative blood vessels). The infiltrating tumor cells are CD3 negative (F), CD5 positive (G), CD10 negative (H) and bcl-6 weakly positive (I). Bcl-2 was positive and MUM1/IRF4 was negative (not illustrated). Cyclin D1 shows variable nuclear positivity (J) and MIB1 (K) shows a proliferation fraction of 40–50%. (L) An H&E stain from the patient's bone marrow trephine biopsy showing involvement by mantle cell lymphoma (MCL).

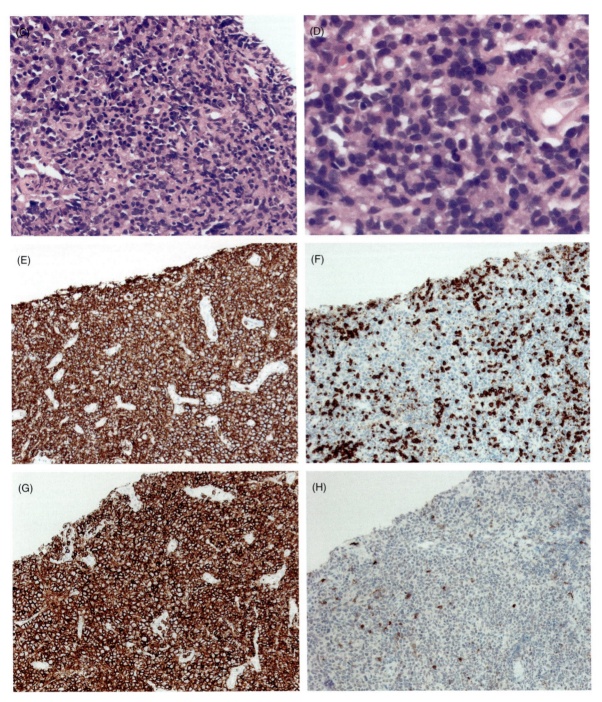

Illustrative case (cont.)

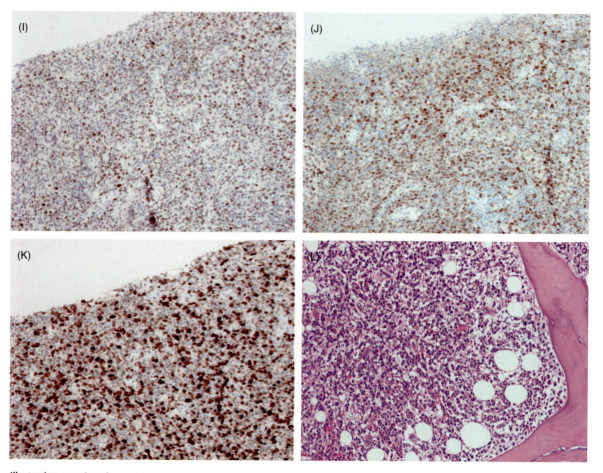

(I)

(J)

(K)

(L)

Illustrative case (cont.)

Burkitt lymphoma

Core biopsies from Burkitt lymphoma (BL) show a diffuse monomorphic infiltrate of small to medium-sized lymphoid cells with rounded nuclei and small basophilic nucleoli (Fig. 7.1A–D). The cells have a small or moderate amount of deeply basophilic cytoplasm in which lipid vacuoles may be seen in cytological preparations. The infiltrate is dense and the tumor cells are closely packed to form apparently cohesive or almost syncytial sheets. The cells of BL are often described as showing "squared-off" borders where the cells have retracted from each other, but this may not be visible in core biopsies. Mitotic figures are frequent in BL, but it is the apoptoses that are more important; almost all cases will show apoptotic nuclear debris, usually in significant amounts (Fig. 7.1B–D). This debris is often concentrated in the cytoplasm of scattered macrophages that interrupt the sheets of tumor cells to give the "starry sky" appearance.[1–4] However, not all cases show this pattern, and this starry sky morphology can be found in tumors other than BL, so on its own should not be considered as a diagnostic feature. There are three main clinical subtypes of BL – endemic BL, sporadic BL and immunodeficiency-associated BL. The morphological findings in all subtypes are similar, although the prototypic features are more associated with the endemic subtype.

Immunohistochemistry

Most cases of BL show a typical immunohistochemical staining pattern.[5] The tumor cells express B-lineage markers (CD20, CD79a, PAX5) (Fig. 7.1E) and are negative for CD3 and CD5. They have a germinal center phenotype and express CD10 and bcl-6 (Fig. 7.1F,G) but show negative or very weak expression of bcl-2 (Fig. 7.1H,I). MUM1/IRF4 is usually negative (Fig. 7.1J), but some cases are positive. MIB1 shows a very high proliferation fraction, with almost all the tumor cells expressing this marker

(Fig. 7.1K). Epstein–Barr virus (EBV) is important in the etiology of BL, particularly in endemic BL, and EBER staining is positive in 25–40% of all cases (Fig. 7.1L).[6] Well-fixed cases can show membrane staining with IgM and light chain restriction. Immunohistochemistry for MYC protein shows nuclear positivity in 80–90% of tumor cells in BL, but a subset of diffuse large B cell lymphomas can also show this pattern; many of the latter also have a c-myc translocation.[7] Fluorescence in-situ hybridization (FISH) studies are valuable in BL, as the finding of a c-myc translocation in the absence of other chromosomal changes will support the diagnosis.[8,9] Table 7.1 summarizes the immunohistochemical staining of BL.

Differential diagnosis

1. Diffuse large B cell lymphoma (DLBCL). This condition is the major differential diagnosis of BL.[10,11] Whilst most cases of BL show typical morphology, there are examples with increased nuclear pleomorphism and/or more prominent nucleoli. In addition, there are cases of DLBCL where the tumor cells are monomorphic and show with frequent mitoses and apoptoses (including a starry sky pattern). At the genetic level, approximately 10% of DLBCL will also show a c-myc translocation, although this is often combined with other abnormalities such as bcl-6 or bcl-2 rearrangements.[12,13] There are cases that cannot be definitively assigned to either category, and the World Health Organization recognizes an intermediate ("gray zone") lymphoma – "B cell lymphoma unclassifiable with features intermediate between diffuse large B cell lymphoma and Burkitt lymphoma."[14] In practice cases with broadly appropriate morphology, a strong germinal center

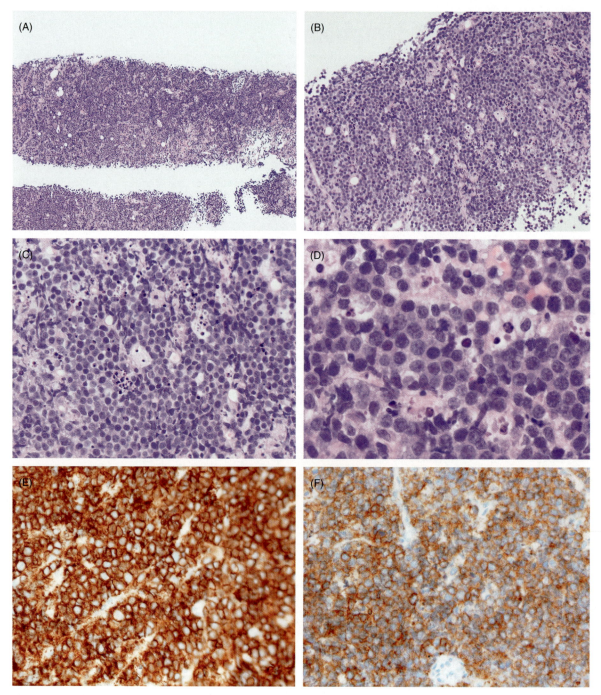

Figure 7.1 Burkitt lymphoma (BL). (A–D) H&E sections from a morphologically typical case of BL. There is a diffuse infiltrate of monomorphic tumor cells interspersed with macrophages containing apoptotic debris giving the "starry sky" appearance. The tumor cells are rounded with minimal cytoplasm and small nucleoli and nuclear debris is prominent (C,D). The tumor cells are CD20 positive (E), CD10 positive (F), bcl-6 positive (G) and MUM1/IRF4 negative (H). Bcl-2 can be weakly positive (I), but most BL cases are bcl-2 negative (J). MIB1 shows a proliferation fraction that approaches 100% (K). Image (L) is a positive EBER staining from an Epstein–Barr virus (EBV) positive case of BL.

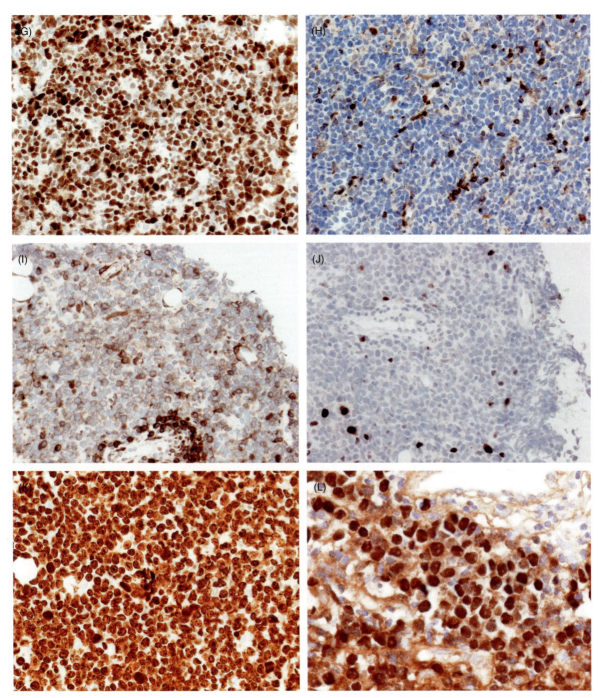

Figure 7.1 (cont.)

phenotype, a weak or negative bcl-2 and a proliferation fraction of close to 100% should be put into the BL category and FISH studies should be carried out. This will give the clinicians the opportunity to consider the use of BL-type chemotherapy and will prevent a patient potentially missing out on the best treatment.[5]

Table 7.1 Panel of antibodies useful in the diagnosis of BL

Antibody	Specificity	Utility
CD20	Glycosylated phosphoprotein expressed on the surface of B cells	Confirms B lineage (may be negative in patients treated with rituximab)
CD79a	B cell antigen receptor alpha chain	Alternative B lineage marker (unaffected by rituximab)
PAX5	B cell marker – protein regulator expressed in early stages of B cell differentiation	Alternative B lineage marker (unaffected by rituximab) – nuclear stain
CD3	T cell marker – part of the protein complex associated with the T cell receptor	Stains background reactive T lymphocytes – relatively low numbers in BL (in contrast with DLBCL)
MIB1	Detects Ki67 nuclear protein associated with cell proliferation	Very high in BL (95–100%)
CD10	Common ALL antigen positive in germinal center B cells	Positive in BL
Bcl-6	Transcription factor expressed in the nuclei of germinal center B cells	Positive in BL
Bcl-2	Apoptosis regulator over-expressed in most cases of follicular lymphoma	Typically negative in BL, but many cases show weak positivity and some cases are strongly positive
MUM1/IRF4	B cell proliferation and differentiation marker	Frequently negative in BL, but some cases are positive
MYC protein	*C-myc* encoded protein involved in cell proliferation and differentiation	Nuclear positivity in 80–90% of BL tumor cells; also positive in a subset of DLBCL
Cyclin D1	Cyclin protein involved in cell cycle regulation	Negative in BL. Nuclear positivity in MCL
TdT (Terminal deoxynucleotidyl transferase)	DNA polymerase expressed in immature lymphoid cells	Negative in BL – positive in B (and T) lymphoblastic leukemia/lymphoma
EBER	Epstein–Barr encoded viral RNA	Positive in a subset of BL cases; more common in endemic and immunodeficiency-associated BL

Abbreviations: ALL, acute lymphoblastic leukemia; BL, Burkitt lymphoma; DLBCL, diffuse large B cell lymphoma; MCL, mantle cell lymphoma.

2. Lymphoblastic leukemia/lymphoma (LBL). The monomorphic sheets of blasts seen in LBL can mimic the tumor cells of BL. LBL may show a starry sky pattern and a high proliferation fraction. However, TdT is negative in BL and most cases of LBL are bcl-2 positive.

3. Mantle cell lymphoma (MCL). The blastoid variant of MCL can resemble BL, especially where MIB1 is high. CD5 and cyclin D1 staining will identify MCL and are negative in BL. Note that SOX11 can be positive in BL.[15]

Burkitt lymphoma: problems and pitfalls of core biopsies

- Cellular morphology is variable in core biopsies, particularly where fixation is sub-optimal. The sheets of tumor cells may be less cohesive than in an excision biopsy, and the starry sky pattern may be subtle or absent.

- As mentioned above, some cases of BL show increased nuclear pleomorphism and larger nucleoli. In the past many of these case were categorized as "atypical BL," but the genetic profile of these cases was found to resemble that of standard BL and it is now accepted that the condition shows a spectrum of cellular morphology. However, there still are cases where a clear distinction from DLBCL or a "gray zone" lymphoma is not possible.

- Bcl-2 staining can be problematic in BL. Although typical cases show negative or only weakly positive staining with this antibody, some cases are strongly bcl-2 positive.[16] Such cases are still categorized as BL if all other features are compatible with this diagnosis, and there is evidence of a *c-myc* translocation in the absence of *bcl-2* or *bcl-6* rearrangements.[17]

References

1. Wright DH. Burkitt's lymphoma: a review of the pathology, immunology, and possible etiologic factors. *Pathol Annu* 1971;**6**:337–363.

2. Burkitt DP. The discovery of Burkitt's lymphoma. *Cancer* 1983;**51**:1777–1786.

3. Magrath IT. African Burkitt's lymphoma. History, biology, clinical features, and treatment. *Am J Pediatr Hematol Oncol* 1991;**13**:222–246.

4. Yustein JT, Dang CV. Biology and treatment of Burkitt's lymphoma. *Curr Opin Hematol* 2007;**14**:375–381.

5. Bellan C, Stefano L, Giulia de F, Rogena EA, Lorenzo L. Burkitt lymphoma versus diffuse large B-cell lymphoma: a practical approach. *Hematol Oncol* 2010;**28**:53–56.

6. Schwemmle M, Clemens MJ, Hilse K, et al. Localization of Epstein–Barr virus-encoded RNAs EBER-1 and EBER-2 in interphase and mitotic Burkitt lymphoma cells. *Proc Natl Acad Sci U S A* 1992;**89**:10292–10296.

7. Green TM, Nielsen O, de Stricker K, et al. High levels of nuclear MYC protein predict the presence of MYC rearrangement in diffuse large B-cell lymphoma. *Am J Surg Pathol* 2012;**36**:612–619.

8. Haralambieva E, Banham AH, Bastard C, et al. Detection by the fluorescence in situ hybridization technique of MYC translocations in paraffin-embedded lymphoma biopsy samples. *Br J Haematol* 2003;**121**:49–56.

9. Hecht JL, Aster JC. Molecular biology of Burkitt's lymphoma. *J Clin Oncol* 2000;**18**:3707–3721.

10. Chuang SS, Ye H, Du MQ, et al. Histopathology and immunohistochemistry in distinguishing Burkitt lymphoma from diffuse large B-cell lymphoma with very high proliferation index and with or without a starry-sky pattern: a comparative study with EBER and FISH. *Am J Clin Pathol* 2007;**128**:558–564.

11. de Leval L, Hasserjian RP. Diffuse large B-cell lymphomas and Burkitt lymphoma. *Hematol Oncol Clin North Am* 2009;**23**:791–827.

12. Berger R, Bernheim A. Cytogenetics of Burkitt's lymphoma-leukaemia: a review. *IARC Sci Publ* 1985;**60**:65–80.

13. Kornblau SM, Goodacre A, Cabanillas F. Chromosomal abnormalities in adult non-endemic Burkitt's lymphoma and leukemia: 22 new reports and a review of 148 cases from the literature. *Hematol Oncol* 1991;**9**:63–78.

14. Hoeller S, Copie-Bergman C. Grey zone lymphomas: lymphomas with intermediate features. *Adv Hematol* 2012;**2012**:460801.

15. Dictor M, Ek S, Sundberg M, et al. Strong lymphoid nuclear expression of SOX11 transcription factor defines lymphoblastic neoplasms, mantle cell lymphoma and Burkitt's lymphoma. *Haematologica* 2009;**94**:1563–1568.

16. Pervez S, Raza MQ, Mirza A, Pal A. Strong BCL2 expression in Burkitt lymphoma is not uncommon in adults. *Indian J Pathol Microbiol* 2011;**54**:290–293.

17. Seegmiller AC, Garcia R, Huang R, et al. Simple karyotype and bcl-6 expression predict a diagnosis of Burkitt lymphoma and better survival in IG-MYC rearranged high-grade B-cell lymphomas. *Mod Pathol* 2010;**23**:909–920.

Illustrative case: Burkitt lymphoma

7

Illustrative case

History: Male aged 47. Newly diagnosed as human immunodeficiency virus (HIV) positive. Biopsy of left axillary lymph node.

Comments: The core biopsy here shows a closely packed sheet of monomorphic tumor cells with interspersed macrophages. There is a significant amount of apoptotic debris, both within the macrophage cytoplasm and amidst the tumor cells. The infiltrating cells show rounded nuclear outlines and small multiple nucleoli. CD20 and CD79a are positive, confirming a B cell lineage. CD3 is negative on the tumor cells and shows a relatively low content of reactive background T cells. CD10 and bcl-6 are positive and bcl-2 shows weak cytoplasmic positivity. MUM1 is completely negative and MIB1 shows a proliferation fraction that approaches 100%. The tumor cells are EBER positive. Fluorescence in-situ hybridization (FISH) detected a *c-myc* translocation.

This is a good example of an immunodeficiency-associated BL. The immunohistochemical findings are typical; the tumor cells are B cell and have a germinal center phenotype. There is a paucity of background T cells, weak staining with bcl-2, negative MUM1/IRF4, a MIB1 fraction of 100% and EBER positivity. Most cases of immunodeficiency-associated BL arise in the setting of HIV, as seen here. The lymphoma in this case was the clinical presentation of the patient's HIV infection.

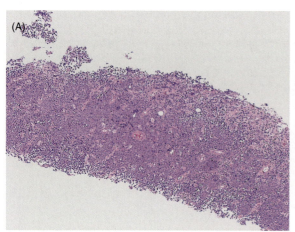 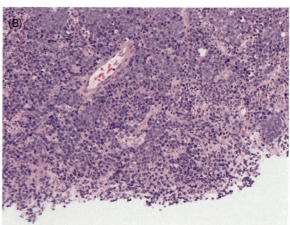

Illustrative case (A–D) H&E stains show the typical morphological features of Burkitt lymphoma (BL). Low power shows a dense monomorphic cellular infiltrate with some pale histiocytic cells giving a "starry sky" appearance (A). At higher powers (B–D) the tumor cells are uniform and rounded with small nucleoli and minimal cytoplasm. Prominent apoptotic debris is seen in macrophages and the tumor cells show frequent mitotic figures (D). The cells are B cells and are CD20 positive (E) and CD3 negative (F). The tumor has a germinal center phenotype – CD10 and bcl-6 are positive (G,H). Bcl-2 shows some very weak membrane positivity (I), MUM1 is negative (J), and MIB1 shows a high proliferation fraction – almost all the tumor cells are positive (K). This case was Epstein–Barr virus (EBV)-positive; EBER staining showed nuclear positivity in the tumor cells (L).

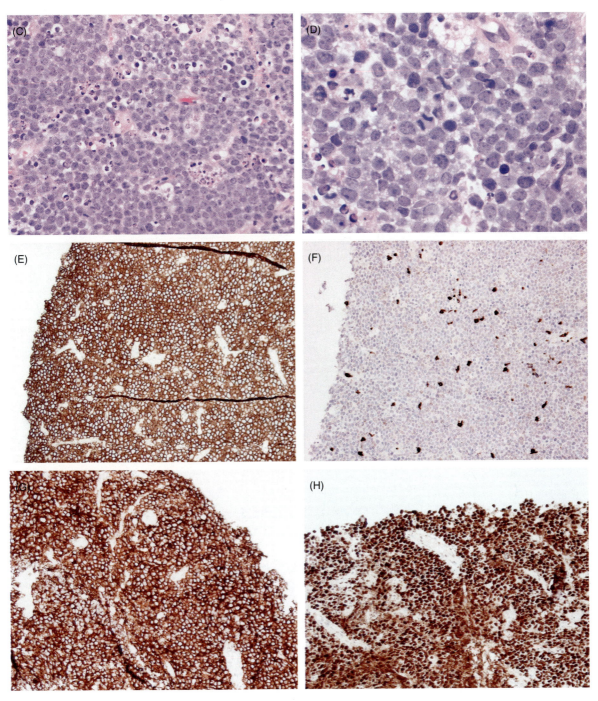

Illustrative case (cont.)

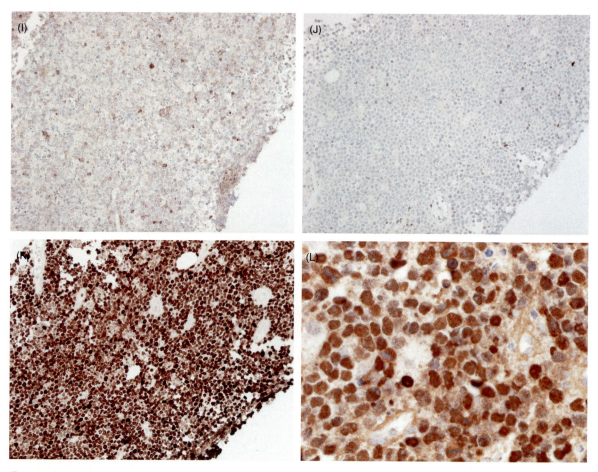

Illustrative case (cont.)

Marginal zone lymphoma and lymphoplasmacytic lymphoma

Marginal zone lymphoma (MZL) can be seen in core biopsies in a number of settings. Whilst some biopsies may come from mucosa-associated lymphoid tissue (MALT) sites such as salivary gland or thyroid, the majority will be from lymph nodes. The latter can contain nodal MZL or nodes involved by a local extra-nodal MZL of MALT. It may not be possible to distinguish nodal and extranodal MZL in needle core biopsies.[1–3]

The infiltrate of MZL is usually diffuse, although some biopsies show a vague nodularity that relates to infiltration or replacement of underlying follicles (see below). Where the biopsy comes from a MALT site, residual epithelium may be present and occasionally lymphoepithelial lesions can be seen. In some cases there may be residual lymphoid follicles with reactive germinal centers. The typical MZL consists of sheets of small lymphoid cells with slightly irregular dark nuclei that have absent or small nucleoli (Fig. 8.1A–D). These cells resemble the normal centrocytes seen in germinal centers and are referred to as "centrocyte-like." Other MZL cases contain larger cells with pale cytoplasm and lighter, more lobulated nuclei – "monocytoid" cells (Fig. 8.1E).[4,5] Marginal zone lymphoma can also show a variable degree of plasmacytic differentiation. Some cases will contain a sub-population of cells with a plasmablastic or plasmacytoid appearance and in others there are mature plasma cells. The MZL cell types – centrocytic, monocytoid and plasmacytic – are not mutually exclusive, and two or all three can be found in some cases. Marginal zone lymphoma with plasmacytic differentiation can resemble lymphoplasmacytic lymphoma (LPL). Although LPL is predominantly a bone marrow disease, nodal disease does occur and there is a morphological and immunophenotypic overlap with MZL.[6,7]

Marginal zone lymphoma cells are positive with all the B lineage antibodies (Fig. 8.1F) and are negative with CD3 and CD5 T cell markers (Fig. 8.1G). Germinal center cell markers are negative, although bcl-6 can show some positivity (see below; Fig. 8.1H,I), and bcl-2 is positive (Fig. 8.1J).[8] MUM1/IRF4 is usually negative in centrocyte-like cells but will be expressed by plasmacytic cells or mature plasma cells. CD138 will stain a mature plasma cell component. CD43 is positive in up to 50% of MZL cases, but can also stain other B cell neoplasms and so is not a specific marker.[9,10] IgM is typically positive (but IgG and IgA-positive cases are seen) and IgD is negative (Fig. 8.1K,L).[11,12] The latter contrasts with chronic lymphocytic leukemia/small lymphocytic lymphoma (CLL/SLL) and follicular lymphoma (FL), which normally express IgD. With ideal fixation the cells of MZL will show light chain restriction, with cytoplasmic light chain staining in the plasmacytic component. The proliferation fraction with MIB1 (Fig. 8.1M) is variable but it is usually low (less than 40%).

Differential diagnosis

1. Both MZL and LPL fall into the small B cell lymphoma category which includes FL, mantle cell lymphoma (MCL) and CLL/SLL.[13] In ideal cases, FL will be identified by the presence of neoplastic follicles and CLL/SLL will show typical proliferation centers, but the morphology in core biopsies is rarely definitive, and immunohistochemistry is usually required to distinguish these entities. In addition, reactive (bcl-2 negative) follicles can be seen in association with nodal or extranodal MZL, and can add to the diagnostic complexity. Table 6.1 in Chapter 6 lists the panel of antibodies used in this setting. In practice the most common differential of MZL is FL, so CD10, bcl-6 and CD21 are most useful. The B cells in MZL/LPL are CD5 negative and do not express cyclin D1.

2. Biopsies from a plasma cell neoplasm (PCN) such as a plasmacytoma or deposit of plasma cell myeloma can mimic cases of MZL with extreme

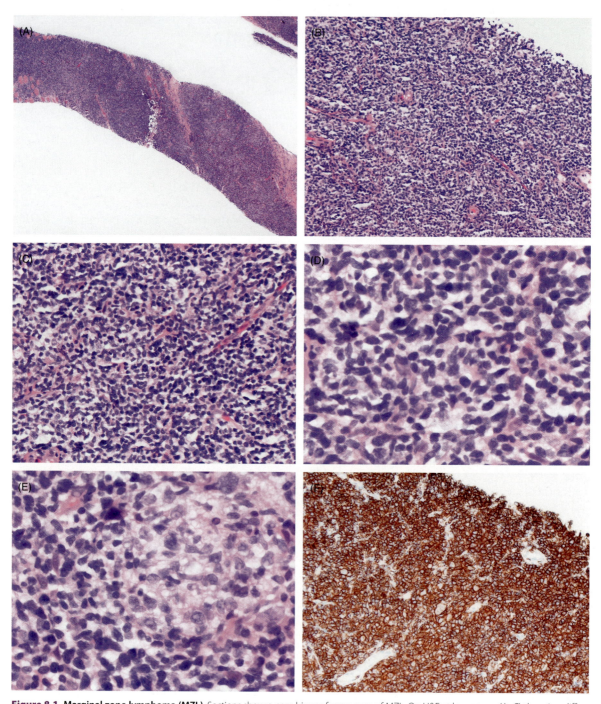

Figure 8.1 Marginal zone lymphoma (MZL). Sections show a core biopsy from a case of MZL. On H&E at low power (A–C) there is a diffuse infiltrate of small lymphoid cells. At higher power there is a mixture of cells with irregular ("centrocyte-like") nuclear outlines, small or absent nucleoli and little cytoplasm (D) and clusters of larger cells with a more monocytoid appearance (E). The latter cells have larger slightly lobulated nuclei with small nucleoli and prominent pale cytoplasm. The tumor cells are CD20 positive (F). CD5 (G) stains admixed T cells but is negative on the tumor cells. CD10 is negative (H), bcl-6 shows some patchy weak positivity (I), and bcl-2 is positive (J). The tumor cells are IgM positive (K) and IgD negative (L) and MIB1 shows a low overall proliferation fraction of approximately 5% (M).

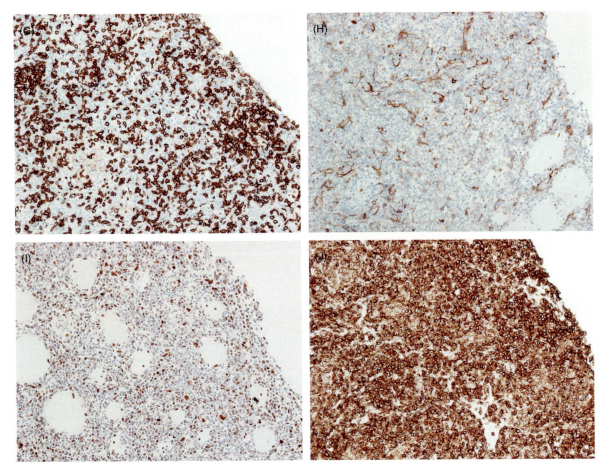

Figure 8.1 (cont.)

plasma cell differentiation. The cells in a PCN are normally CD138 positive and will not express CD20 or PAX5, although some neoplastic plasma cells can show aberrant CD20 staining. Neoplastic plasma cells may also express CD56 or cyclin D1, which is not a feature of MZL or LPL, and IgM expression is very rare in PCN. The two entities cannot always be distinguished, and on occasion it is necessary to report a case as representing "either a PCN or marginal zone lymphoma showing extreme plasma cell differentiation."[14]

3. Although the morphology and phenotype of MZL and LPL can overlap, molecular studies for MYD88 L265P mutation can enable the distinction of these entities. The MYD88 L265P mutation is a highly sensitive marker for LPL and can be carried out on paraffin-fixed tissue.[15,16]

Marginal zone lymphoma: problems and pitfalls of core biopsies

- There are no specific immunohistochemical markers for MZL – the diagnosis is normally one of exclusion. It should be noted that CD43 staining is not specific for MZL as this antibody stains a number of B cell lymphomas.

- CD23 staining is not specific for CLL/SLL; some cases of MZL or LPL are CD23 positive and very rare examples express CD5.

- Although most cases of MZL and LPL are IgM positive, this is not universal. An absence of staining with IgD is more useful than IgM positivity.

- Although bcl-6 is a marker of germinal center cells, weak or patchy positivity can be seen in MZL, LPL and other small B cell lymphomas.

81

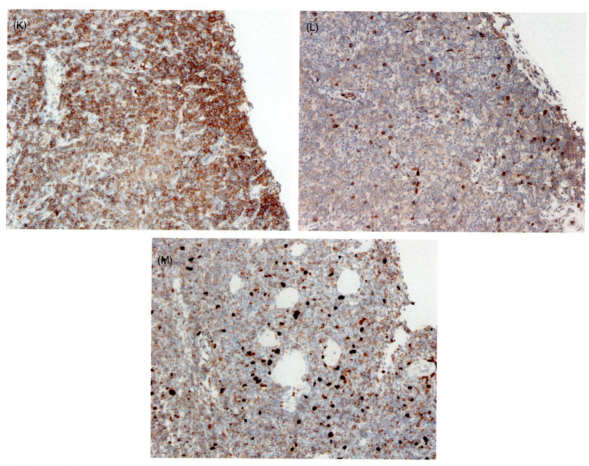

Figure 8.1 (cont.)

- Colonization or replacement of pre-existing lymphoid follicles can result in an apparent follicular structure. When combined with weak bcl-6 staining and bcl-2 positivity this feature may lead to an erroneous diagnosis of FL.[17]

References

1. Dierlamm J, Pittaluga S, Wlodarska I, et al. Marginal zone B-cell lymphomas of different sites share similar cytogenetic and morphologic features. *Blood* 1996;**87**:299–307.

2. de Wolf-Peeters C, Pittaluga S, Dierlamm J, Wlodarska I, Van Den Berghe H. Marginal zone B-cell lymphomas including mucosa-associated lymphoid tissue type lymphoma (MALT), monocytoid B-cell lymphoma and splenic marginal zone cell lymphoma and their relation to the reactive marginal zone. *Leuk Lymphoma* 1997;**26**:467–478.

3. Nathwani BN, Drachenberg MR, Hernandez AM, Levine AM, Sheibani K. Nodal monocytoid B-cell lymphoma (nodal marginal-zone B-cell lymphoma). *Semin Hematol* 1999;**36**:128–138.

4. Thieblemont C, Davi F, Noguera ME, Brière J. Non-MALT marginal zone lymphoma. *Curr Opin Hematol* 2011;**18**:273–279.

5. Arcaini L, Lucioni M, Boveri E, Paulli M. Nodal marginal zone lymphoma: current knowledge and future directions of an heterogeneous disease. *Eur J Haematol* 2009;**83**:165–174.

6. Berger F, Traverse-Glehen A, Felman P, et al. Clinicopathologic features of Waldenstrom's macroglobulinemia and marginal zone lymphoma: are they distinct or the same entity? *Clin Lymphoma* 2005;**5**:220–224.

7. Lin P, Molina TJ, Cook JR, Swerdlow SH. Lymphoplasmacytic lymphoma and other non-marginal zone lymphomas with plasmacytic differentiation. *Am J Clin Pathol* 2011;**136**:195–210.

8. Salama ME, Lossos IS, Warnke RA, Natkunam Y. Immunoarchitectural patterns in nodal marginal zone

B-cell lymphoma: a study of 51 cases. *Am J Clin Pathol* 2009l;**132**:39–49.

9. Lai R, Weiss LM, Chang KL, Arber DA. Frequency of CD43 expression in non-Hodgkin lymphoma. A survey of 742 cases and further characterization of rare CD43[+] follicular lymphomas. *Am J Clin Pathol* 1999;**111**:488–494.

10. Salama ME, Lossos IS, Warnke RA, Natkunam Y. Immunoarchitectural patterns in nodal marginal zone B-cell lymphoma: a study of 51 cases. *Am J Clin Pathol* 2009;**132**:39–49.

11. Spencer J, Perry ME, Dunn-Walters DK. Human marginal-zone B cells. *Immunol Today* 1998;**19**:421–426.

12. Maes B, De Wolf-Peeters C. Marginal zone cell lymphoma – an update on recent advances. *Histopathology* 2002;**40**:117–126.

13. Swerdlow SH. Small B-cell lymphomas of the lymph nodes and spleen: practical insights to diagnosis and pathogenesis. *Mod Pathol* 1999;**12**:125–140.

14. Hussong JW, Perkins SL, Schnitzer B, Hargreaves H, Frizzera G. Extramedullary plasmacytoma. A form of marginal zone cell lymphoma? *Am J Clin Pathol* 1999;**111**:111–116.

15. Treon SP, Xu L, Yang G, et al. MYD88 L265P somatic mutation in Waldenström's macroglobulinemia. *N Engl J Med* 2012;**367**:826–833.

16. Xu L, Hunter ZR, Yang G, et al. MYD88 L265P in Waldenström macroglobulinemia, immunoglobulin M monoclonal gammopathy, and other B-cell lymphoproliferative disorders using conventional and quantitative allele-specific polymerase chain reaction. *Blood* 2013;**121**:2051–2058.

17. Kojima M, Nakamura S, Murase T, et al. Follicular colonization of nodal marginal-zone B-cell lymphoma resembling follicular lymphoma: report of six cases. *Int J Surg Pathol* 2005;**13**:73–78.

8 Illustrative case: Marginal zone lymphoma and lymphoplasmacytic lymphoma

Illustrative case

History: Male aged 67. Core biopsy of mass in the soft tissue of right chest wall. Possible soft tissue tumor?

Comments: This core biopsy shows no lymph node structures and is composed of diffuse sheets of small to medium-sized lymphoid cells, which show a striking histological appearance. There is a mixture of small centrocyte-like cells and larger cells that have pale nuclei with single eosinophilic nucleoli. These latter cells resemble small plasmablasts. In addition there are cells with distended eosinophilic cytoplasm in which the nucleus is displaced to the periphery. The infiltrate is B cell and is CD20 positive but CD138 shows a significant sub-population with plasmacytic differentiation. There is cytoplasmic expression of IgM and kappa light chain. CD5, CD10, bcl-6, cyclin D1, CD56, CD23 and IgD (not illustrated) were negative. MIB1 shows a moderate proliferation fraction (approximately 40%).

This biopsy shows a lesion that occupies the borderline between marginal zone lymphoma with plasmacytic differentiation and lymphoplasmacytic lymphoma. There is a mixture of CD20-positive B cells and CD138-positive plasma cells. The cells with plasmablastic morphology and those with eosinophilic cytoplasm make up the CD138-positive subset. The eosinophilic material in the cytoplasm is immunoglobulin, and stains with IgM and kappa light chain. Such cytoplasmic distension by immunoglobulin can give the cells a "signet ring" appearance. Dutcher bodies are not seen here. The patient had Stage IV disease with involvement of the chest wall and testis. He was treated as if he had an extranodal marginal zone lymphoma.

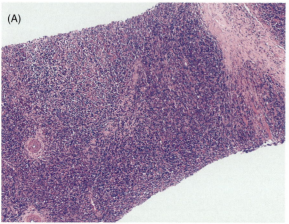

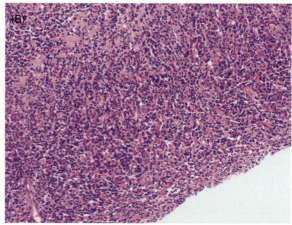

Illustrative case (A–E) H&E sections show a core biopsy with a diffuse infiltrate of small and medium-sized cells, some of which have striking eosinophilic cytoplasm. The higher power sections (D,E) show a mixture of small lymphocytes with irregular dark nuclei, medium-sized cells with paler nuclei and single eosinophilic nucleoli and larger cells in which the nucleus is displaced to the side by eosinophilic cytoplasmic contents. Immunostaining shows that the infiltrating cells are CD20 positive (F) although there are a significant number of admixed CD3-positive T cells (G). CD138 staining (H) shows plasmacytic differentiation in a sub-population of the tumor cells. The tumor cells show cytoplasmic expression of IgM (I) and kappa light chain (J); lambda staining is negative (K). MIB1 shows a moderate proliferation fraction (L).

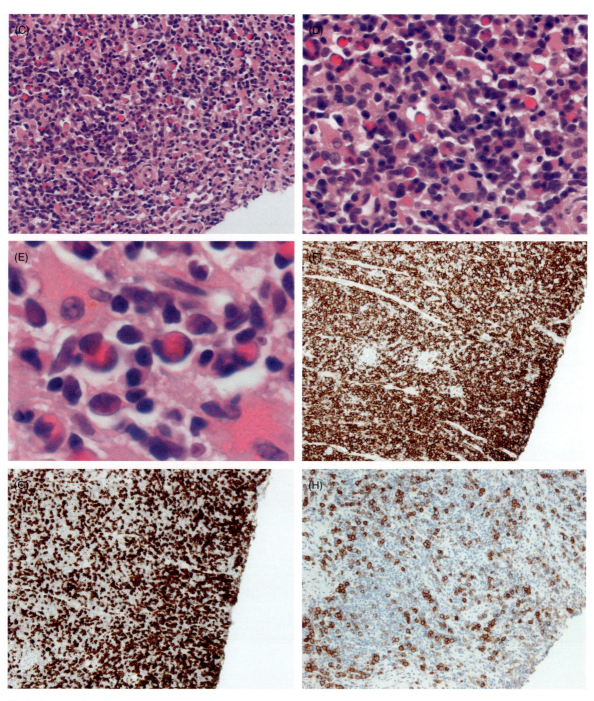

Illustrative case (cont.)

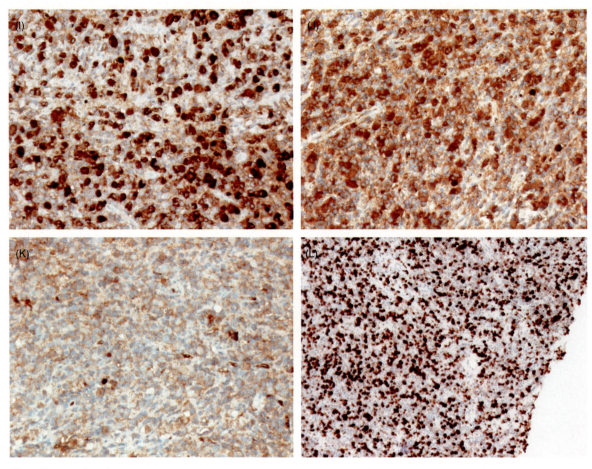

Illustrative case (cont.)

Chapter 9

Diffuse large B cell lymphoma

Diffuse large B cell lymphoma (DLBCL) is relatively commonly seen in needle core biopsies. As a group, DLBCL includes a wide range of lymphomas, both subtypes of the condition and closely related entities.[1] Lymphomas in this group include T cell/histiocyte rich large B cell lymphoma,[2] Epstein–Barr virus (EBV) positive DLBCL of the elderly,[3] primary mediastinal large B cell lymphoma (PMLBCL),[4] intravascular large B cell lymphoma,[5] ALK-positive large B cell lymphoma[6] and plasmablastic lymphoma.[7] The histological appearances are protean, but most cases consist of a diffuse sheet of pleomorphic large lymphoid cells (Figs 9.1A–D, 9.2A–D). The tumor cells usually have moderate amounts of cytoplasm and

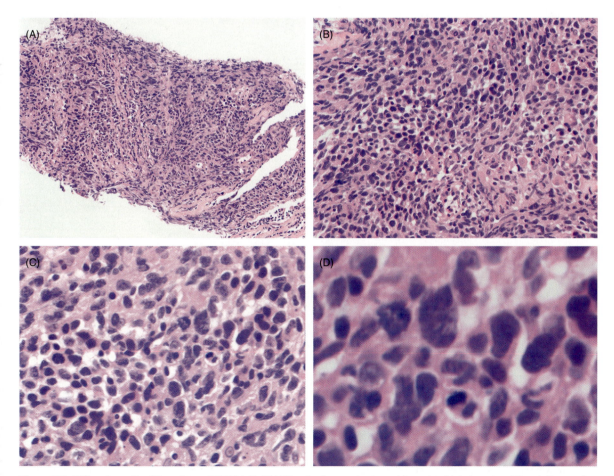

Figure 9.1 Diffuse large B cell lymphoma (DLBCL). (A–D) H&E stains from a short core biopsy in which there is a diffuse infiltrate of pleomorphic atypical cells. Although the morphology is not obviously that of lymphoma, CD20 is positive (E); both cytokeratin and S100 staining were negative. The tumor cells express CD10 (F), bcl-6 (G), and MUM1/IRF4 (H). MIB1 shows a proliferation fraction of approximately 50% (I).

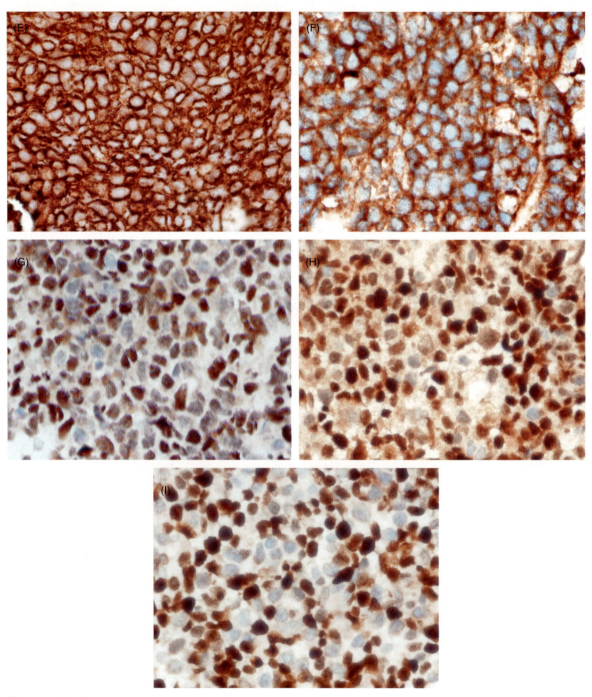

Figure 9.1 (cont.)

show irregular nuclei with prominent eosinophilic, often multiple nucleoli. The cells may morphologically resemble germinal center centroblasts, can have an immunoblastic appearance (Fig. 9.2D), may show pale polylobated nuclei or can have a highly anaplastic appearance (Fig. 9.1A–D). The latter may require immunohistochemistry to confirm a B cell lymphoid lineage. Mitoses are common and areas of necrosis are not infrequent (Fig. 9.2A). Cases may express immunoglobulin heavy and light chains.

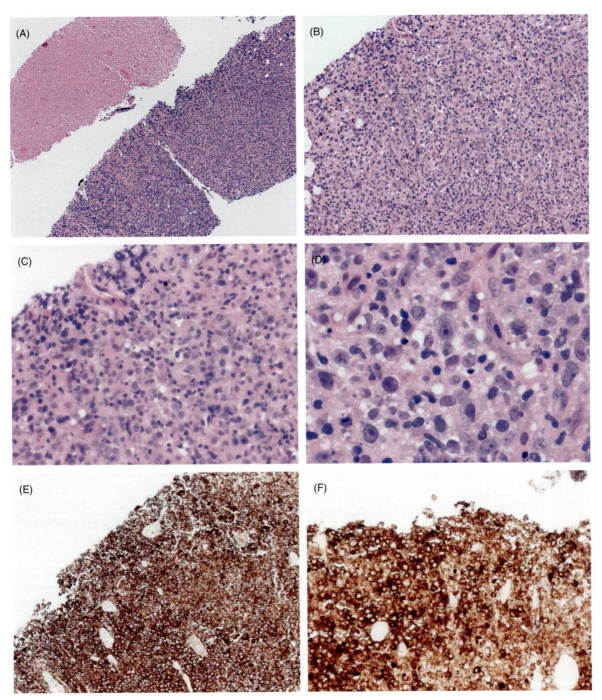

Figure 9.2 Diffuse large B cell lymphoma (DLBCL). (A) Low power H&E showing a short necrotic core and a longer core infiltrated by tumor. At higher power (B–D) the tumor is made up of a diffuse sheet of large lymphoid cells with pale cytoplasm and prominent nucleoli. CD20 staining is positive both on the viable tumor cells (E) and in the necrotic region (F). CD3 shows an interspersed population of reactive T cells (G). CD10 is negative (H), bcl-6 is weakly positive (I), MUM1/IRF4 is focally positive (J) and bcl-2 is positive (K). This tumor is Epstein–Barr virus (EBV) positive; the tumor cells show nuclear staining with EBER in-situ hybridization (L). MIB1 shows a proliferation fraction of 50–60% (M).

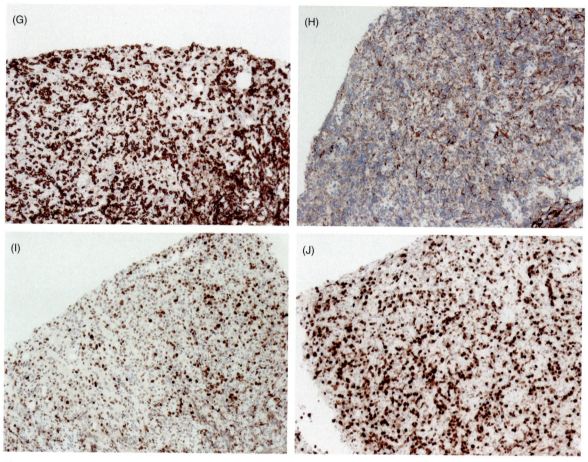

Figure 9.2 (cont.)

Immunohistochemistry

Immunohistochemistry is critical both in identifying a tumor as DLBCL and in assigning cases into prognostic subgroups. CD20 is positive in most cases (Figs 9.1E, 9.2E,F), but some are negative so other B cell lineage markers (CD79a, PAX5, CD19 and CD22) may be required. CD3 will normally show a significant content of reactive/background T cells (Fig. 9.2G) and MIB1 shows proliferation fraction of at least 40% (Figs 9.1I, 9.2M). There is variable expression of germinal center cell markers CD10 and bcl-6 (Figs 9.1F,G, 9.2H,I), and of bcl-2 and MUM1/IRF4 (Figs 9.1H, 9.2J,K). Other specific antibodies are helpful in the identification of DLBCL variants or related entities; CD23 is frequently positive in PMLBCL,[8] EBER in-situ hybridization is positive in the EBV-positive DLBCL lymphoma of the elderly (Fig. 9.2L) and ALK1 staining is positive in ALK-positive large

B cell lymphoma. A list of antibodies useful in the diagnosis of DLBCL is provided in Table 9.1.

Diffuse large B cell lymphoma is a clinically heterogeneous disease, and the pathological findings can contribute to patient risk stratification. The initial approach to identifying prognostic subtypes involved using a combination of germinal center cell markers and MUM/IRF4 to divide cases into germinal center and non-germinal center subtypes.[9] Although the algorithm used for this division (Fig. 9.3) correlates to some extent with gene expression profiling studies,[10,11] the outcome has been shown to be of limited clinical significance in patients treated with rituximab.[12] Because of this the germinal center/non-germinal center phenotypic distinction is no longer considered accurate enough for treatment decisions. Current evidence supports a key role for bcl-2 and MYC. Diffuse large B cell lymphoma with combined *bcl-2* and *c-myc*

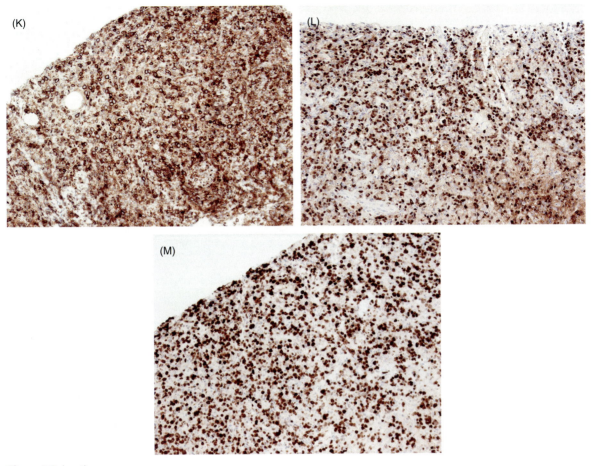

(K)

(L)

(M)

Figure 9.2 (cont.)

translocations ("double hit" lymphomas) are associated with a worse prognosis when treated with conventional R-CHOP chemotherapy.[13] Bcl-2 protein expression has been shown to be an independent predictor of outcome in DLBCL,[14,15] and recent studies have confirmed that high MYC protein expression is also an adverse prognostic feature in DLBCL.[16] MYC protein expression also correlates with *c-myc* gene status.[17] Significantly, concurrent immunohistochemical expression of both MYC and bcl-2 proteins in DLBCL is associated with inferior overall and progression-free survival.[18–20] Where immunohistochemical expression of both MYC and bcl-2 is accompanied by "double hit" cytogenetic translocations the prognosis is extremely poor.[20] For these reasons it is important that the pathological assessment of DLBCL includes immunohistochemistry and fluorescence in-situ hybridization

(FISH) for both *c-myc* and *bcl-2*. Cases with adverse "double hit" cytogenetics are considered for more aggressive chemotherapy from the outset.

Differential diagnosis

1. Classical Hodgkin lymphoma (CHL). The pleomorphic large cells of DLBCL may resemble Hodgkin/Reed–Sternberg cells, and in some cases the large cells are CD30 positive. In contrast to CHL, the neoplastic cells in DLBCL usually form sheets, are CD15 negative and are CD45 positive. Expression of both OCT-2 and BOB1 (see Table 3.1) is rare in CHL and common in DLBCL. It is not always possible to assign a lymphoma to either category, and the World Health Organization recognizes an intermediate ("gray zone") entity – B cell lymphoma

Table 9.1 Extended table of antibodies useful in the diagnosis of DLBCL and closely related entities

Antibody	Specificity	Utility
CD20	Glycosylated phosphoprotein expressed on the surface of B cells	Confirms B lineage (may be negative in patients treated with rituximab)
CD79a	B cell antigen receptor alpha chain	Alternative B lineage marker (unaffected by rituximab)
PAX5	B cell marker – protein regulator expressed in early stages of B cell differentiation	Alternative B lineage marker (unaffected by rituximab) – nuclear stain
CD3	T cell marker – part of the protein complex associated with the T cell receptor	Stains background reactive T lymphocytes
CD5	T cell surface glycoprotein	Positive in a subset of DLBCL
CD10	Common ALL antigen positive in germinal center B cells	Part of prognostic algorithm to determine germinal center/non-germinal center phenotype
Bcl-6	Transcription factor expressed in the nuclei of germinal center B cells	Part of prognostic algorithm to determine germinal center/non-germinal center phenotype
MUM1/ IRF4	B cell proliferation and differentiation marker	Part of prognostic algorithm to determine germinal center/non-germinal center phenotype
Bcl-2	Apoptosis regulator over-expressed in most cases of follicular lymphoma	Independent prognostic marker in DLBCL
MYC protein	*C-myc* encoded protein involved in cell proliferation and differentiation	Independent prognostic marker in DLBCL. May indicate underlying *c-myc* translocation
Cyclin D1	Cyclin protein involved in cell cycle regulation, over-expressed in mantle cell lymphoma	Marks a subset of DLBCL; negative staining in CD5-positive DLBCL excludes pleomorphic variant of mantle cell lymphoma
CD23	B cell low affinity IgE receptor	Commonly positive in primary mediastinal large B cell lymphoma
EBER	Epstein–Barr encoded viral RNA	Positive in a subset of DLBCL and in EBV-positive DLBCL of the elderly
CD30	Cell membrane protein in the tumor necrosis factor receptor family; marks activated lymphoid cells	Positive in a subset of DLBCL; commonly expressed in primary mediastinal large B cell lymphoma (80%)
ALK1	Anaplastic lymphoma kinase; tyrosine kinase receptor over-expressed in anaplastic large cell lymphoma	Positive in the rare ALK-positive large B cell lymphoma
MIB1	Recognizes the Ki67 antigen – a nuclear protein associated with cell proliferation	Determines the growth fraction of DLBCL which to some extent correlates with the clinical course and is prognostic for survival and recurrence

Abbreviations: ALL, acute lymphoblastic leukemia; DLBCL, diffuse large B cell lymphoma; EBV, Epstein–Barr virus.

unclassifiable with features intermediate between diffuse large B cell lymphoma and classical Hodgkin lymphoma.[21]

2. Pleomorphic mantle cell lymphoma (MCL). This variant of MCL contains large pleomorphic cells with prominent nucleoli and morphologically resembles DLBCL. CD5, cyclin D1 and SOX11 staining are helpful here, although both CD5-positive and cyclin D1-positive DLBCL are recorded (see below). FISH for the CCND1 translocation should be negative in DLBCL.

3. Burkitt lymphoma (BL). This differential is discussed in Chapter 7. Cases of DLBCL with more monomorphic cells, a high proliferation rate and a germinal center phenotype with negative bcl-2 staining can resemble BL. DLBCL may also harbor a *c-myc* translocation, although this is usually in combination with other chromosomal abnormalities. As with CHL, not all cases can be assigned to either BL or DLBCL categories, and an intermediate entity is also recognized in this area (B cell lymphoma unclassifiable with features intermediate between diffuse large B cell lymphoma and BL).[22]

4. Non-lymphoid tumors. The more anaplastic forms of DLBCL can resemble metastatic carcinoma,

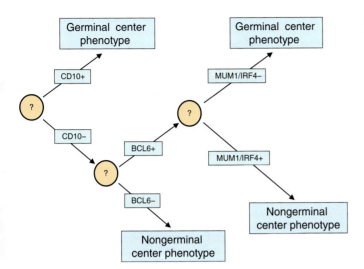

melanoma, or germ cell tumor. Positive verification of a B cell origin will confirm the diagnosis of DLBCL, but initial panels may need to include cytokeratins, melanoma markers (S100, HMB45, melan-A) and germ cell markers (PLAP, OCT-3/4, CD117, CD30).

5. Peripheral T cell lymphoma, not otherwise specified (PTCL-NOS). The morphology of PTCL-NOS can closely resemble that of DLBCL. Immunohistochemistry will normally confirm the lineage of the tumor cells. Bear in mind that PTCL-NOS can show loss of pan-T cell markers and some cases of DLBCL will lack CD20 (or other pan-B markers) so in extended panels should be used when lineage is not clear.

6. Anaplastic large cell lymphoma (ALCL). Highly anaplastic examples of DLBCL will often express CD30 and may be negative with some B lineage markers. ALCL may lack pan-T markers and can occasionally show aberrant expression of B cell markers such as CD20. EMA expression can be seen in both conditions. Extended B cell panels will usually identify cases of DLBCL. ALCL can be identified by strong expression of cytotoxic markers, and by ALK1 staining in the ALK-positive form.

7. Infectious mononucleosis (IM). The EBV-driven B cell proliferation in IM can resemble DLBCL (see Chapter 2). The mixed cellular infiltrate in IM (both B cell and T cell) and the clinical features will usually enable the distinction of these conditions. EBER staining in IM is in both large transforming cells and small lymphocytes, whereas only the large cells stain in an EBV-positive large B cell lymphoma.

8. Histiocytic sarcoma and myeloid sarcoma. These rare conditions can show similar morphology to that of DLBCL. Histiocytic sarcoma is usually pleomorphic and resembles an anaplastic DLBCL, whereas myelosarcoma is composed of more monomorphic cells. Immunohistochemistry will not identify any staining with B cell markers and will show variable positivity with histiocytic and myeloid antibodies (CD68, MPO, CD13, CD11c, CD163).

Diffuse large B cell lymphoma: problems and pitfalls of core biopsies

- Cell size. Despite the name, not all DLBCLs are made up of large cells. This seems to be more common in core biopsies, so it is not uncommon to come across a diffuse infiltrate of medium-sized or even small cells that show nuclear pleomorphism and a high mitotic rate. These cases can be difficult to distinguish from conditions such as follicular lymphoma with a diffuse pattern. Whilst a high MIB1 fraction may be helpful (and clinical features can contribute), sometimes it is necessary to produce an indefinite report and/or request a repeat biopsy.
- Interfollicular DLBCL.[23] Where the core biopsy only shows focal disease in the interfollicular regions it can be difficult to distinguish DLBCL from a prominent paracortical reaction.

93

Expression of germinal center cell markers in cells outwith the germinal centers suggests a neoplastic process, and light chain restriction or detection of a clone by polymerase chain reaction (PCR) can confirm the diagnosis of DLBCL.

- CD20-negative DLBCL. Some cases of DLBCL are CD20 negative, and some patients will have had rituximab treatment. Use of other pan-B cell markers can help here. Note that cases towards the plasmablastic end of the spectrum will lose both CD20 and PAX5; CD79a expression should be retained.
- A subset of DLBCL cases express CD5.[24] Mantle cell lymphoma should be excluded by cyclin D1 and SOX11 staining together with FISH for the CCND1 translocation.
- A subset of DLBCL cases can express cyclin D1.[25] These are usually CD5 and SOX11 negative and will lack the CCND1 translocation.
- Some cases of DLBCL can show highly unusual morphology. Examples include tumors composed of spindle-shaped cells that can resemble a sarcoma,[26] tumors with myxoid stromal changes that can resemble mucinous adenocarcinoma, and tumors with a prominent granulomatous reaction. Despite the odd morphology, the tumor cells will express B cell markers and can be identified by immunohistochemistry.

References

1. Menon MP, Pittaluga S, Jaffe ES. The histological and biological spectrum of diffuse large B-cell lymphoma in the World Health Organization classification. *Cancer J* 2012;**18**:411–420.

2. Tousseyn T, De Wolf-Peeters C. T cell/histiocyte-rich large B-cell lymphoma: an update on its biology and classification. *Virchows Arch* 2011;**459**:557–563.

3. Adam P, Bonzheim I, Fend F, Quintanilla-Martínez L. Epstein–Barr virus-positive diffuse large B-cell lymphomas of the elderly. *Adv Anat Pathol* 2011;**18**:349–355

4. Martelli M, Ferreri AJ, Johnson P. Primary mediastinal large B-cell lymphoma. *Crit Rev Oncol Hematol* 2008;**68**:256–263.

5. Orwat DE, Batalis NI. Intravascular large B-cell lymphoma. *Arch Pathol Lab Med* 2012;**136**:333–338.

6. Beltran B, Castillo J, Salas R, et al. ALK-positive diffuse large B-cell lymphoma: report of four cases and review of the literature. *J Hematol Oncol* 2009;**2**:11.

7. Hsi ED, Lorsbach RB, Fend F, Dogan A. Plasmablastic lymphoma and related disorders. *Am J Clin Pathol* 2011;**136**:183–194.

8. Calaminici M, Piper K, Lee AM, Norton AJ. CD23 expression in mediastinal large B-cell lymphomas. *Histopathology* 2004;**45**:619–624.

9. Barrans SL, Carter I, Owen RG, et al. Germinal center phenotype and bcl-2 expression combined with the International Prognostic Index improves patient risk stratification in diffuse large B-cell lymphoma. *Blood* 2002;**99**:1136–1143.

10. Berglund M, Thunberg U, Amini RM, et al. Evaluation of immunophenotype in diffuse large B-cell lymphoma and its impact on prognosis. *Mod Pathol* 2005;**18**:1113–1120.

11. Rosenwald A, Staudt LM. Gene expression profiling of diffuse large B-cell lymphoma. *Leuk Lymphoma* 2003;44 Suppl 3:S41–47.

12. Hong J, Park S, Park J, et al. Evaluation of prognostic values of clinical and histopathologic characteristics in diffuse large B-cell lymphoma treated with rituximab, cyclophosphamide, doxorubicin, vincristine, and prednisolone therapy. *Leuk Lymphoma* 2011;**52**:1904–1912.

13. Johnson NA, Savage KJ, Ludkovski O, et al. Lymphomas with concurrent BCL2 and MYC translocations: the critical factors associated with survival. *Blood* 2009;**114**:2273–2279.

14. Shivakumar L, Armitage JO. Bcl-2 gene expression as a predictor of outcome in diffuse large B-cell lymphoma. *Clin Lymphoma Myeloma* 2006;**6**:455–457.

15. Iqbal J, Meyer PN, Smith LM, et al. BCL2 predicts survival in germinal center B-cell-like diffuse large B-cell lymphoma treated with CHOP-like therapy and rituximab. *Clin Cancer Res* 2011;**17**:7785–7795.

16. Kluk MJ, Chapuy B, Sinha P, et al. Immunohistochemical detection of MYC-driven diffuse large B-cell lymphomas. *PLoS One* 2012;**7**:e33813.

17. Tapia G, Lopez R, Muñoz-Mármol AM, et al. Immunohistochemical detection of MYC protein correlates with MYC gene status in aggressive B cell lymphomas. *Histopathology* 2011;**59**:672–678.

18. Johnson NA, Slack GW, Savage KJ, et al. Concurrent expression of MYC and BCL2 in diffuse large B-cell lymphoma treated with rituximab plus cyclophosphamide, doxorubicin, vincristine, and prednisone. *J Clin Oncol* 2012;**30**:3452–3459.

19. Horn H, Ziepert M, Becher C, et al.; German High-Grade Non-Hodgkin Lymphoma Study Group. MYC status in concert with BCL2 and BCL6 expression predicts outcome in diffuse large B-cell lymphoma. *Blood* 2013;**121**:2253–2263.

20. Hu S, Xu-Monette ZY, Tzankov A, et al. MYC/BCL2 protein coexpression contributes to the inferior survival of activated B-cell subtype of diffuse large B-cell lymphoma and demonstrates high-risk gene expression signatures: a report from The International DLBCL Rituximab-CHOP Consortium Program. *Blood* 2013;**121**:4021–4031.

21. Carbone A, Gloghini A, Aiello A, Testi A, Cabras A. B-cell lymphomas with features intermediate between distinct pathologic entities. From pathogenesis to pathology. *Hum Pathol* 2010;**41**:621–631.

22. Hoeller S, Copie-Bergman C. Grey zone lymphomas: lymphomas with intermediate features. *Adv Hematol* 2012;**2012**:460801.

23. Yamauchi A, Ikeda J, Nakamichi I, et al.; Osaka Lymphoma Study Group. Diffuse large B-cell lymphoma showing an interfollicular pattern of proliferation: a study of the Osaka Lymphoma Study Group. *Histopathology* 2008;**52**:731–737.

24. Salles G, de Jong D, Xie W, et al. Prognostic significance of immunohistochemical biomarkers in diffuse large B-cell lymphoma: a study from the Lunenburg Lymphoma Biomarker Consortium. *Blood* 2011;**117**:7070–7078.

25. Rodriguez-Justo M, Huang Y, Ye H, et al. Cyclin D1-positive diffuse large B-cell lymphoma. *Histopathology* 2008;**52**:900–903.

26. Carbone A, Gloghini A, Libra M, et al. A spindle cell variant of diffuse large B-cell lymphoma possesses genotypic and phenotypic markers characteristic of a germinal center B-cell origin. *Mod Pathol* 2006;**19**:299–306.

9 Illustrative cases: Diffuse large B cell lymphoma

Illustrative case 1

History: Female aged 24. Presented with fever, night sweats, chest pain and an anterior mediastinal mass. The clinical differential diagnosis included lymphoma, metastatic carcinoma and a germ cell tumor.

Comments: Histology shows a diffuse infiltrate of cells with lymphoid morphology. There is a sclerotic background which separates small groups of tumor cells to give a "packeted" appearance. The tumor cells are medium-sized to large with irregular, often pale, nuclei and multiple small nucleoli. CD20 is positive, confirming a B cell lesion. CD3 shows a small number of reactive T cells. The tumor cells express CD10, bcl-6 and bcl-2 and are strongly CD23 positive. MIB1 shows a proliferation fraction of (80–90%). CD30, cytokeratin and MUM1/IRF4 are negative; TdT and EBER were also negative.

The clinical and morphological features are those of primary mediastinal large B cell lymphoma. The packeted appearance on histology is typical for this lesion, as is the expression of CD23. Although this

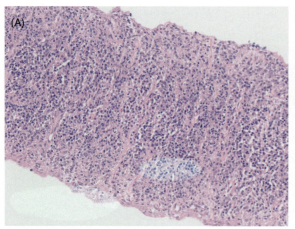
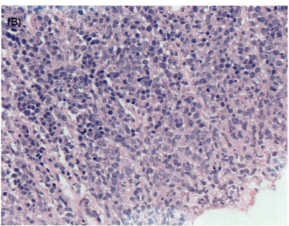

Illustrative case 1 (A–D) H&E sections show a diffuse infiltrate of large lymphoid cells. There is some background fibrosis giving a hint of tumor cell "packeting," and the cells have pale nuclei and small nucleoli (D). CD20 is positive (E) and CD3 shows scattered background T cells (F). Both CD30 staining (G) and cytokeratin staining (H) are negative. The lymphoma is CD10 positive (I), bcl-6 positive (J), MUM1/IRF4 negative (K) and bcl-2 positive (L). MIB1 shows a high proliferation fraction (80–90%, M) and the tumor cells show widespread CD23 positivity (N).

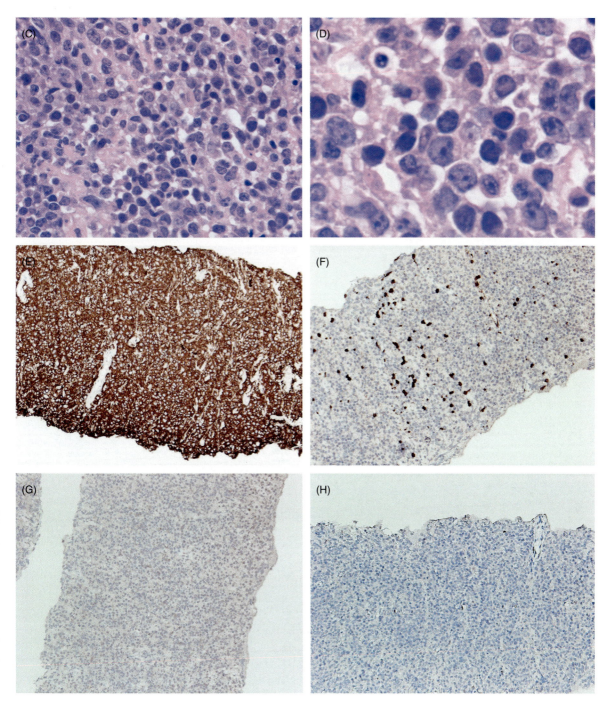

Illustrative case 1 (cont.)

case was CD30 negative, most (80%) are positive. CD10 expression, as seen here, is less common in this entity. This tumor shows a gene expression profile that is distinct from that of diffuse large B cell lymphoma, not otherwise specified (DLBCL-NOS), and shares some features with classical Hodgkin lymphoma. The lesion is considered to arise from thymic B cells, and occasionally thymic epithelial remnants can be seen within the tumor, although this is extremely rare in core biopsies.

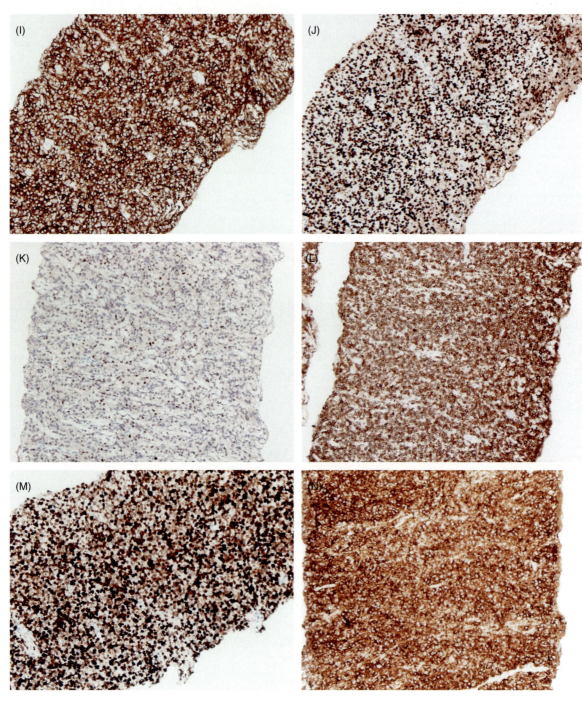

Illustrative case 1 (cont.)

Illustrative case 2

History: Male aged 74 with known sarcoid. Infiltration of femur with pathological fracture and multiple enlarged lymph nodes in right groin. Needle biopsy of groin node.

Comments: The biopsy shows a diffuse infiltrate consisting of sheets of histiocytes forming confluent granulomas admixed with collections of large pleomorphic lymphoid cells. CD20 staining shows the lymphoid

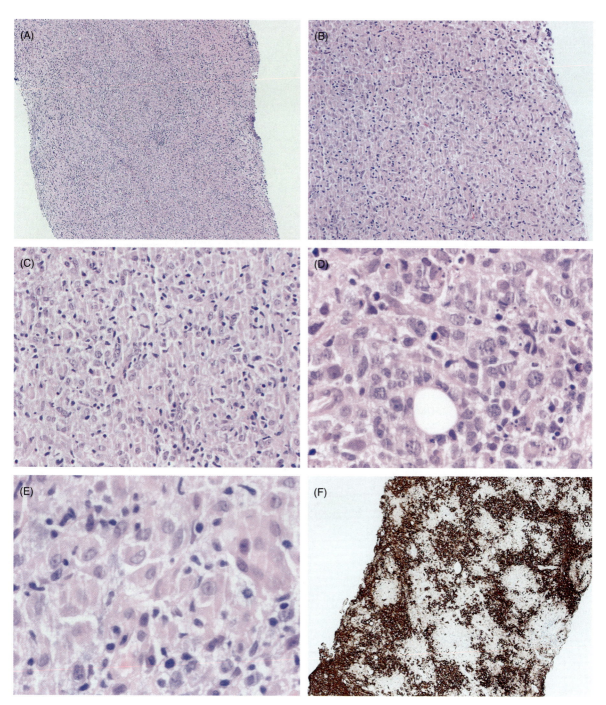

Illustrative case 2 (A–F) H&E stains show sheets of pale histiocytes and admixed lymphoid cells. At low power (A–C) the neoplastic cells are not immediately obvious. Higher power (D) shows large pleomorphic lymphoid cells with the morphological features of diffuse large B cell lymphoma. A high power view of the histiocytes is shown in image (E). Immunohistochemical staining clarifies the cellular populations present. Images (F) and (G) show the CD20-positive tumor cell population. Image (H) is a CD3 stain showing a background T cell population. The collections of histiocytes are positive with CD11c (I) and CD68 (KP1, J). The lymphoma cells are CD10 positive (K), bcl-6 positive (L) and MUM1/IRF4 positive (M). Bcl-2 is positive (N) and MIB1 shows a proliferation fraction of 60–70% in the tumor cells (O).

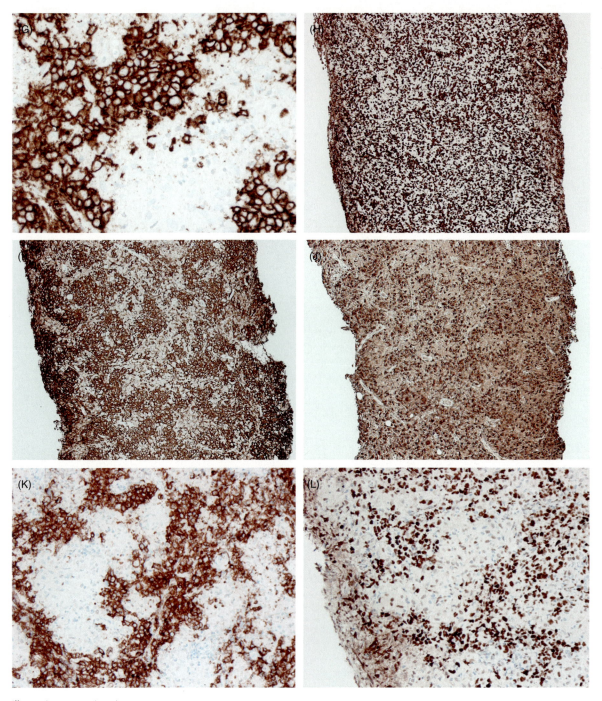

Illustrative case 2 (cont.)

population, with clear "gaps" for the histiocytic/granulomatous reaction. The histiocytes are CD11c and CD68 positive. CD3 shows numerous background T cells and CD10 positivity in the tumor cells indicates a germinal center phenotype.

This diffuse large B cell lymphoma is arising in a patient with sarcoid, and there is a marked granulomatous reaction in this biopsy, presumably a response to the tumor. Many lymphomas can excite a granulomatous reaction (classical Hodgkin

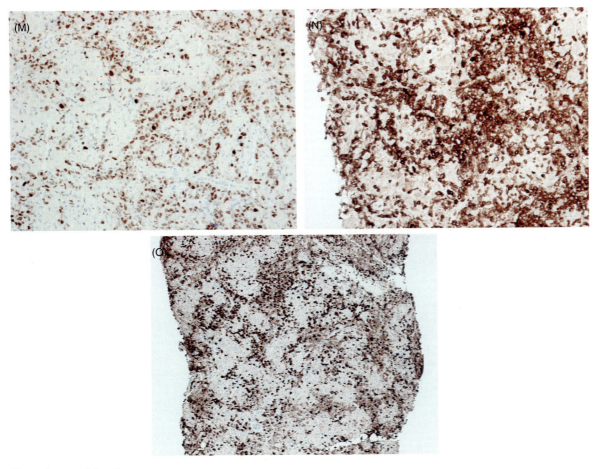

Illustrative case 2 (cont.)

lymphoma probably being the most frequent), even in patients without a systemic granulomatous condition such as sarcoidosis. When faced with a biopsy showing sheets or collections of histiocytes, the morphology should be carefully assessed for the presence of an associated lymphoma, and an appropriate immunohistochemical panel should be used to characterize any abnormal lymphoid infiltrate.

Illustrative case 3

History: Male aged 26. Jaundiced with bulky coeliac axis and retroperitoneal lymph nodes and an enlarged spleen. Core biopsy from coeliac axis lymph nodes.

Comments: Unlike most diffuse large B cell lymphoma where there is a sheet of tumor cells, this biopsy shows a mixed infiltrate consisting of scattered, separate, large pleomorphic cells on a background of small lymphocytes. The large cells show marked nuclear pleomorphism with prominent nucleoli and even some mummified forms. They stain as B cells and express bcl-6; the small background lymphocytes are T cells. CD30 is negative and almost all of the large cells are positive with MIB1.

This is a typical example of a T cell/histiocyte rich large B cell lymphoma. The neoplastic B cells lie separately and do not form sheets or clusters. There is a prominent T cell background, together with significant histiocyte content (not specifically stained for here). The differential diagnosis of this condition includes both classical Hodgkin lymphoma (the negative CD30 is helpful in excluding this diagnosis) and nodular lymphocyte predominant Hodgkin lymphoma. Note that some angio-immunoblastic T cell lymphomas can contain large B cells and can morphologically resemble T cell/histiocyte rich large B cell lymphoma.

101

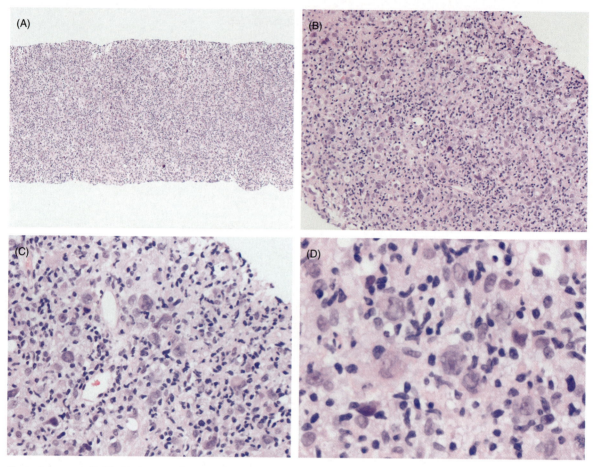

Illustrative case 3 (A–D) H&E shows a diffuse mixed infiltrate with a separated population of large pleomorphic lymphoid cells with prominent nucleoli on a background of small mature lymphocytes. The background lymphocytes are CD3-positive T cells (E), whereas the large cells are B cells and are positive with both CD20 (F) and CD79a (G). The large cells are CD30 negative (H), CD10 negative (I), bcl-6 positive (J) and MUM1/IRF4 negative (K). Bcl-2 is positive in the tumor cells (L), and MIB1 shows that almost all the large cells are in the active phase of the cell cycle (M).

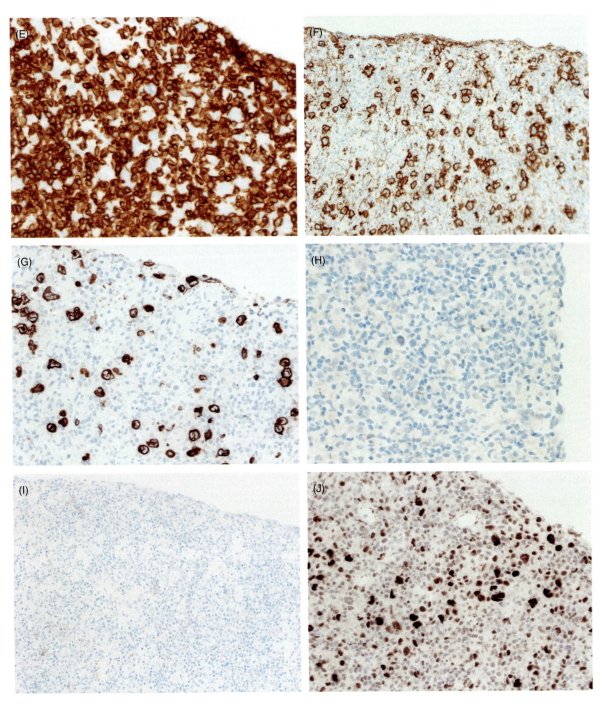

Illustrative case 3 (cont.)

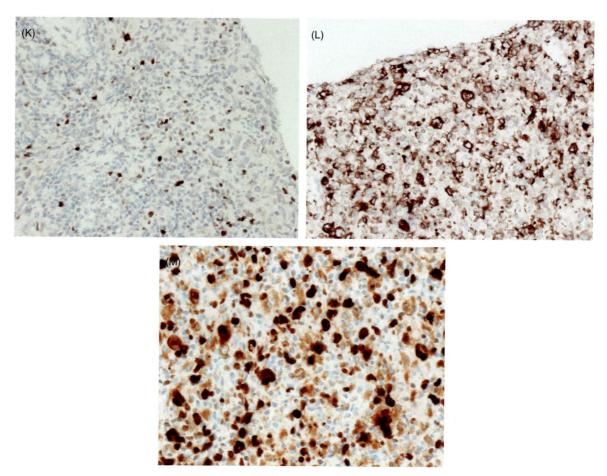

Illustrative case 3 (cont.)

Chapter 10

Chronic lymphocytic leukemia/small lymphocytic lymphoma

Biopsies from cases of chronic lymphocytic leukemia/ small lymphocytic lymphoma (CLL/SLL) show a diffuse infiltrate of small lymphoid cells (Fig. 10.1A–F).[1,2] The leukemic nature of the infiltrate means that the lesion is less destructive than many lymphomas, and some residual nodal structures (intact sinuses or reactive lymphoid follicles) may occasionally be present. The tumor cells usually resemble normal mature lymphocytes, with rounded nuclei, small nucleoli and little cytoplasm (Fig. 10.1C). In practice there is some variability in the cellular morphology, and in some cases the cells have more irregular nuclear outlines and resemble germinal center centrocytes or the cells of mantle cell lymphoma (MCL). In some cases the tumor cells have more cytoplasm and can take on a plasmacytoid appearance suggestive of marginal zone lymphoma (MZL) or lymphoplasmacytic lymphoma (LPL). Although the infiltrate is diffuse, there may be a vague nodularity at low power due to the presence of proliferation centers. These contain larger cells with prolymphocytic or paraimmunoblastic morphology. The prolymphocytes are slightly larger than normal CLL/SLL cells and show multiple small nucleoli (Fig. 10.1D). Paraimmunoblasts are larger still and show round or oval pale nuclei with prominent central eosinophilic nucleoli (Fig. 10.1E,F). Mitotic activity is generally low in CLL/SLL and only slightly raised in the proliferation centers.

The immunophenotype is key to the diagnosis of CLL/SLL.[1–3] The tumor cells express B lineage markers (CD20, CD79a, CD19, CD22, PAX5), are negative with CD3 and are positive with CD5 and CD23 (Fig. 10.1G–J). CD5 is often weaker than on the T cells present, giving a "two tier" staining pattern.[4] Germinal center markers are negative (but see bcl-6 below) and bcl-2 is positive. The tumor cells express surface IgM and IgD and may show light chain restriction.[5] The proliferation centers can be identified with MIB1 or with MUM1/IRF4 which selectively stains paraimmunoblasts (Fig. 10.1K,L).[6]

Differential diagnosis

1. CLL/SLL is another lesion that falls into the well-defined group of small B cell lymphomas.[7,8] This group includes follicular lymphoma (FL), MCL, MZL and LPL. The immunohistochemical panel used to distinguish these entities is summarized in Table 6.1 in Chapter 6. In practice the most common differentials in this group are FL (the proliferation centers can resemble follicles) and MCL (also CD5 positive). FL will express the germinal center cell markers CD10 and bcl-6 and follicular dendritic cell (FDC) networks can be identified with CD21 or CD23. FL is CD5 negative, but can express CD23. MCL will show nuclear positivity with cyclin D1 and SOX11 and will lack proliferation centers.

2. Nodular lymphocyte predominant Hodgkin lymphoma (NLPHL). Occasionally the nodular architecture and collections of small mature lymphocytes in NLPHL can give the morphological impression of CLL/SLL. The findings of typical LP cells together with the lack of CD5 and CD23 staining of the small B lymphocytes will enable the correct identification of this entity.

3. Lymphoblastic leukemia/lymphoma (LBL) can occasionally be composed of small blast cells that resemble CLL/SLL cells. In LBL the tumor cells are less mature and show a higher proliferation rate. Expression of TdT is helpful here, and many cases of B-LBL will be CD10 and/or CD34 positive. In addition MIB1 is usually high (over 60%) in most cases of LBL.

Chronic lymphocytic leukemia/small lymphocytic lymphoma: problems and pitfalls of core biopsies

- Although often readily identifiable in excision biopsies, proliferation centers may not be visible in

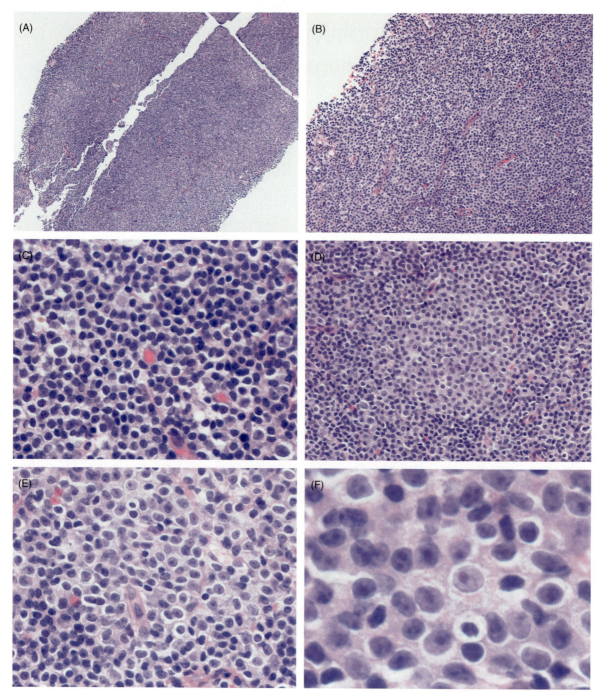

Figure 10.1 Chronic lymphocytic leukemia/small lymphocyte lymphoma (CLL/SLL). (A–F) H&E stains from a case of CLL/SLL with a relatively high content of prolymphocytes and obvious proliferation centers. (A–C) A diffuse infiltrate of small lymphocytes; occasional larger paraimmunoblasts are seen in (C). Image (D) shows a proliferation center consisting of a collection of paler, slightly larger prolymphocytes. At higher power (E,F) the proliferation center contains numerous paraimmunoblasts with central eosinophilic nucleoli. The tumor cells are CD20 positive (G), CD3 negative (H), CD5 positive (I) and CD23 positive (J). Proliferation centers can be identified by MIB1 (K) or by using MUM1/IRF4 to highlight paraimmunoblasts (L).

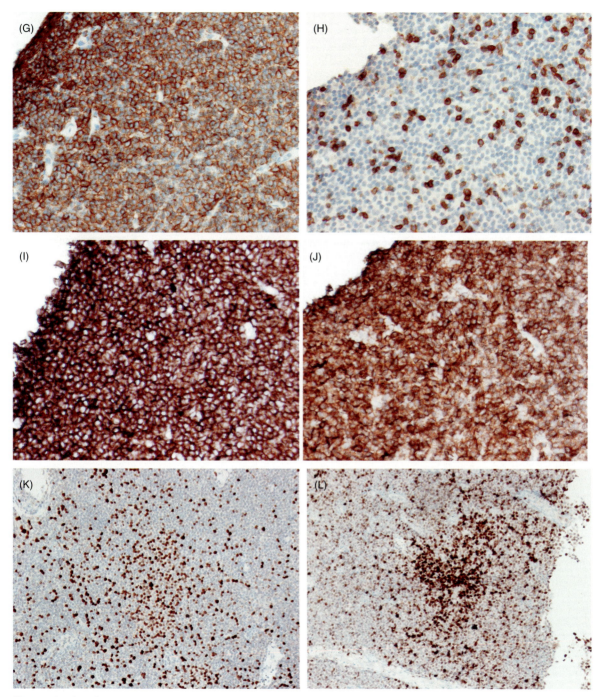

Figure 10.1 (cont.)

core biopsies. The use of both MIB1 and MUM1/
IRF4 staining will help identify these in difficult
cases.[6]

- CD23 is often only focally positive or even
  negative.[9] If the cellular morphology is acceptable,
  where B cell markers and CD5 are clearly positive

and where cyclin D1 is negative, CLL/SLL can be
diagnosed in the absence of CD23 expression.

- CD5 negative CLL/SLL cases are recorded.[10]
  Diagnosis requires a combination of the correct
  clinical picture for CLL/SLL and the pathological
  exclusion of other small B cell lymphomas.

107

- Although bcl-6 is a marker of germinal center cells, weak positive staining is seen in a number of small B cell lymphomas, including CLL/SLL, and does not exclude the diagnosis.
- Transformation to diffuse large B cell lymphoma (DLBCL – Richter syndrome) is seen in 5% of CLL/SLL patients.[11] Pathologically most cases are easy to recognize, but some biopsies can show an "intermediate" picture, with an increase in paraimmunoblasts and a higher MIB1 rate without being an obvious DLBCL. In this setting it is advisable to inform the clinical team that there is a suspicion that the case may be undergoing transformation, and correlation with clinical features (such as raised lactate dehydrogenase [LDH]) may be helpful. There is no evidence that an increase in paraimmunoblasts per se affects prognosis or outcome, so this alone is not grounds for a diagnosis of DLBCL.[12,13]

References

1. Matutes E, Polliack A. Morphological and immunophenotypic features of chronic lymphocytic leukemia. *Rev Clin Exp Hematol* 2000;4:22–47.

2. Inamdar KV, Bueso-Ramos CE. Pathology of chronic lymphocytic leukemia: an update. *Ann Diagn Pathol* 2007;11:363–389.

3. Matutes E, Attygalle A, Wotherspoon A, Catovsky D. Diagnostic issues in chronic lymphocytic leukaemia (CLL). *Best Pract Res Clin Haematol* 2010;23:3–20.

4. Cabezudo E, Carrara P, Morilla R, Matutes E. Quantitative analysis of CD79b, CD5 and CD19 in mature B-cell lymphoproliferative disorders. *Haematologica* 1999;84:413–418.

5. Lewis RE, Cruse JM, Pierce S, Lam J, Tadros Y. Surface and cytoplasmic immunoglobulin expression in B-cell chronic lymphocytic leukemia (CLL). *Exp Mol Pathol* 2005;79:146–150.

6. Soma LA, Craig FE, Swerdlow SH. The proliferation center microenvironment and prognostic markers in chronic lymphocytic leukemia/small lymphocytic lymphoma. *Hum Pathol* 2006;37:152–159.

7. Chen CC, Raikow RB, Sonmez-Alpan E, Swerdlow SH. Classification of small B-cell lymphoid neoplasms using a paraffin section immunohistochemical panel. *Appl Immunohistochem Mol Morphol* 2000;8:1–11.

8. Coelho Siqueira SA, Ferreira Alves VA, Beitler B, Otta MM, Nascimento Saldiva PH. Contribution of immunohistochemistry to small B-cell lymphoma classification. *Appl Immunohistochem Mol Morphol* 2006;14:1–6.

9. DiRaimondo F, Albitar M, Huh Y, et al. The clinical and diagnostic relevance of CD23 expression in the chronic lymphoproliferative disease. *Cancer* 2002;94:1721–1730.

10. Cartron G, Linassier C, Bremond JL, et al. CD5 negative B-cell chronic lymphocytic leukemia: clinical and biological features of 42 cases. *Leuk Lymphoma* 1998;31:209–216.

11. Nakamura N, Abe M. Richter syndrome in B-cell chronic lymphocytic leukemia. *Pathol Int* 2003;53:195–203.

12. Bonato M, Pittaluga S, Tierens A, et al. Lymph node histology in typical and atypical chronic lymphocytic leukemia. *Am J Surg Pathol* 1998;22:49–56.

13. Soma LA, Craig FE, Swerdlow SH. The proliferation center microenvironment and prognostic markers in chronic lymphocytic leukemia/small lymphocytic lymphoma. *Hum Pathol* 2006;37:152–159.

10 Illustrative case: Chronic lymphocytic leukemia/small lymphocytic lymphoma

Illustrative case

History: Female aged 81. FDG-avid lymphadenopathy above and below the diaphragm. Biopsy of right supraclavicular lymph node.

Comments: This core biopsy shows effacement of the normal architecture by a diffuse infiltrate of small lymphoid cells together with non-necrotizing sarcoid-like epithelioid granulomas. The small lymphocytes are monomorphic and show mature morphology; at high power occasional paraimmunoblasts can be identified. The lymphoid infiltrate is CD20 positive, CD3 negative, CD5 positive and CD23 positive. MIB1 shows a low proliferation fraction (less than 10%).

This biopsy shows a case of chronic lymphocytic leukemia/small lymphocytic lymphoma (CLL/SLL) with a sarcoid-like granulomatous reaction to the presence of the tumor. The immunohistochemistry confirms the diagnosis of CLL/SLL, showing that the lymphocytes between the granulomas are CD20, CD5 and CD23 positive. Markers for mantle cell lymphoma (cyclin D1), follicular lymphoma (CD10) and lymphoblastic lymphoma (TdT) were all negative. MIB1 is low and there are no obvious proliferation centers in this biopsy. The case illustrates the importance of assessing the background lymphoid population in all biopsies showing a granulomatous reaction.

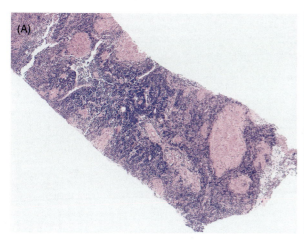
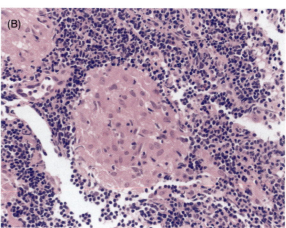

Illustrative case (A–E) H&E sections of this core biopsy show effacement of the normal architecture by a sheet of small lymphoid cells within which are multiple granulomas. The granulomas (D) are non-caseating and are composed of pale epithelioid histiocytes and giant cells. The small lymphoid cells (C,E) show mature morphological features with rounded or slightly irregular nuclei, little cytoplasm and small nucleoli. Occasional paraimmunoblasts contain single, central, larger nucleoli. The tumor cells are CD20 positive (F), CD3 negative (G), CD5 positive (H) and CD23 positive (I). Bcl-2, cyclin D1, CD10 and TdT were negative (not illustrated). MIB1 (J) shows positive scattered cells; no obvious proliferation centers are seen in this specimen.

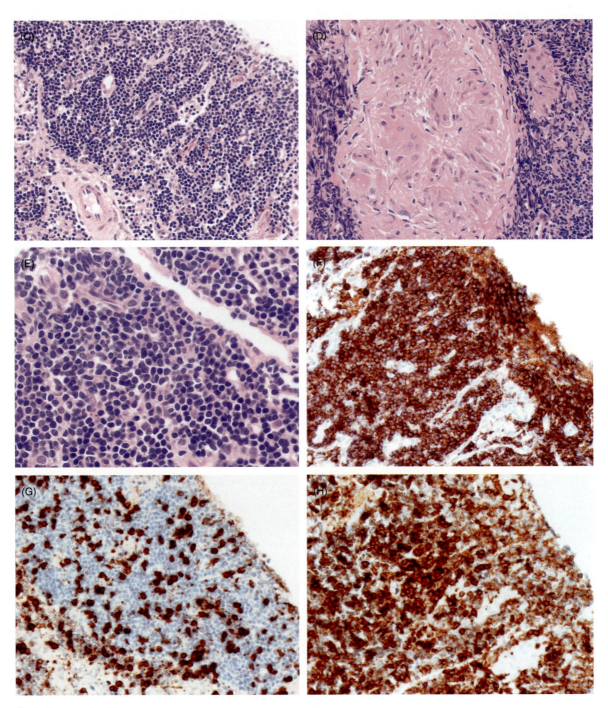

Illustrative case (cont.)

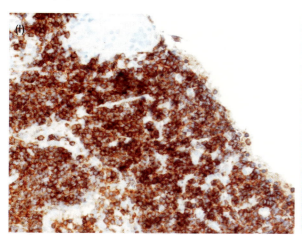

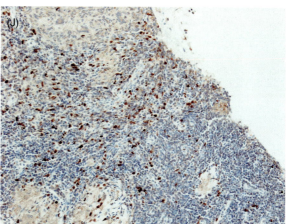

Illustrative case (cont.)

Lymphoblastic leukemia/lymphoma

Lymphoblastic leukemia/lymphoma (LBL) can be of B cell (B-LBL) or T cell (T-LBL) lineage and both lineages show similar morphological features.[1-4] The tumor cells (lymphoblasts) are monomorphic and have small to medium-sized nuclei with little cytoplasm (Fig. 11.1A–E). The nuclei are rounded or slightly irregular and nucleoli, if present, are generally small and inconspicuous (Fig. 11.1D,E). The tumor cells form dense sheets permeating the lymph node, and can take on a nodular appearance when lymphoid follicles are infiltrated. Mitotic activity is prominent, and some cases can show a "starry sky" appearance resembling Burkitt lymphoma. The lymphoblasts are prone to show traction artefact, and nuclear distortion is common, particularly in more fibrous biopsies subjected to trauma during excision (Fig. 11.1A). The tumor cells have a propensity to line up between collagen fibers at the periphery of the node forming a distinctive "Indian file" arrangement (Fig. 11.1C).

Immunohistochemistry

Immunohistochemical investigation involves detection of TdT positivity and determination of the cell lineage.[5] TdT staining is nuclear and shows some variability between individual tumor cells (Fig. 11.1F). Rare TdT negative cases are reported, but these are difficult to diagnose on histopathology alone and will usually require hematological confirmation.[6-9] Lineage markers can be problematic in LBL. B-LBL may not express CD20, and multiple B cell antibodies should be used to confirm the diagnosis (Fig. 11.1G–I).[10] Nuclear staining with PAX5 is probably the most specific marker in this setting (Fig. 11.1I).[11] CD79a is not lineage specific in LBL, and can be positive in T-LBL.[12] Similarly, some cases of B-LBL can express CD5, although CD3 is usually negative (Fig. 11.1J).[13,14] CD10 is positive in the majority of B-LBL cases and in a subset of T-LBLs (Fig. 11.1K).[5] Bcl-6 and MUM1/IRF4 are negative and bcl-2 is usually positive. Markers of precursor cells such as CD34, CD1a and CD99 are often positive, the latter two in T-LBL.[5,15,16] MIB1 generally shows a high mitotic index of over 60% (Fig. 11.1L).[17] Table 11.1 lists the antibodies useful in the diagnosis of LBL.

Differential diagnosis

1. Mantle cell lymphoma (MCL). The cells of the blastoid variant of MCL resemble the lymphoblasts of LBL and both conditions may show high mitotic activity and a degree of nodularity. Immunohistochemistry will enable the distinction of these conditions – MCL is cyclin D1 positive and TdT negative.[18]
2. Follicular lymphoma (FL). The nodularity seen in some cases of LBL can suggest a diagnosis of FL. Although both conditions can be CD10 positive, LBL will express TdT and CD21 staining will show no evidence of follicular dendritic cell networks.
3. Burkitt lymphoma (BL). Both B-LBL and BL are composed of small to medium-sized B cells that can show a high proliferation rate, a "starry sky" pattern and CD10 positivity. TdT staining is critical, and the cells of LBL are usually bcl-6 negative and strongly bcl-2 positive.
4. Myeloid sarcoma. The myeloid blasts in extramedullary deposits of myeloid leukemia can morphologically resemble the lymphoblasts of LBL. TdT can be positive in myeloid sarcoma, but myeloid and myelomonocytic markers (CD117, MPO, CD68) will be positive and lymphoid lineage markers will be negative.

Lymphoblastic leukemia/lymphoma: problems and pitfalls of core biopsies

- The neoplastic cells in T-LBL are morphologically and phenotypically identical to normal cortical thymocytes. A needle biopsy from the thymus gland, or from ectopic thymus tissue, can be

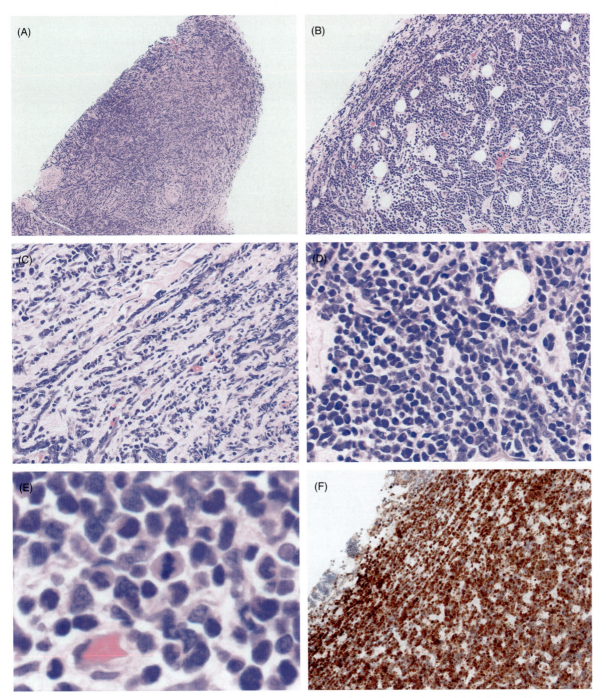

Figure 11.1 B lymphoblastic leukemia/lymphoma (B-LBL). (A–E) H&E stains from a short core biopsy diffusely infiltrated by monomorphic small lymphoid cells. These cells show traction artefact and can be seen to line up between collagen fibers to form "Indian files" (C). At high power (D,E) the cells show hyperchromatic nuclei with irregular nuclear outlines and some molding of nuclei. Nucleoli are small or absent and the cells have a small amount of eosinophilic cytoplasm. Mitotic figures are relatively frequent. TdT (F) is positive in the tumor cells. CD20 (G) shows only scattered positive cells; these may represent residual normal B lymphocytes or focal expression of CD20 by a subset of the tumor cells. In contrast CD79a (H) is strongly positive and PAX5 (I) shows nuclear positivity in the tumor cells. CD3 (J) shows background T cells; the tumor cells are negative. CD10 is strongly positive (K). CD34, bcl-6 and MUM1/IRF4 were negative and bcl-2 was strongly positive. MIB1 shows a high proliferation fraction with 70–80% of tumor cells in cycle (L).

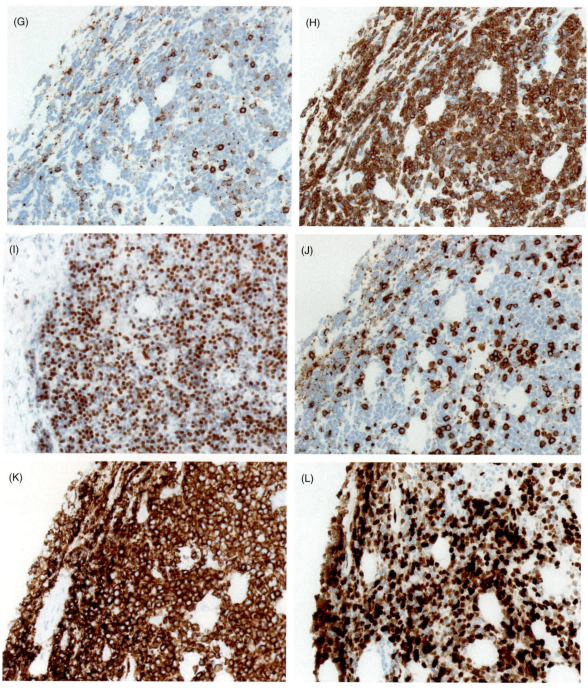

Figure 11.1 (cont.)

mistaken for T-LBL.[19] Close examination should show the presence of larger pale epithelial cells, and possibly Hassall's corpuscles. Cytokeratin staining will reveal the typical thymic epithelial network.

- Traumatic cellular distortion can render the morphology uninterpretable in some biopsies. The distorted cells will usually retain their antigens, so TdT and lymphoid lineage markers will usually enable a diagnosis.

Table 11.1 Extended table of antibodies useful in the diagnosis of lymphoblastic leukemia/lymphoma

Antibody	Specificity	Utility
CD20	Glycosylated phosphoprotein expressed on the surface of B cells	Confirms B cell lineage, but can be negative in B-LBL
CD79a	B cell antigen receptor alpha chain	B lineage marker; can be aberrantly expressed in T-LBL
PAX5	B cell marker – protein regulator expressed in early stages of B cell differentiation	B lineage marker; reliable antibody in B-LBL
CD22	Immune regulatory member of the sialic acid-binding immunoglobulin-type lectins expressed on the surface of B cells	B lineage marker
CD19	Phosphoglycoprotein that forms part of the B cell receptor complex	B lineage marker
CD3	T cell marker – part of the protein complex associated with the T cell receptor	Confirms T cell lineage
CD2	Cell adhesion molecule found on the surface of T cells (and NK cells)	Confirms T cell lineage
CD5	T cell surface glycoprotein	Confirms T cell lineage; can be aberrantly expressed in B-LBL
CD7	Member of immunoglobulin superfamily found on thymocytes and mature T cells	Confirms T cell lineage
TdT (Terminal deoxynucleotidyl transferase)	DNA polymerase expressed in immature lymphoid cells	Nuclear positivity in B and T-LBL (Very rare negative cases)
CD34	Cell surface glycoprotein expressed on early hemopoietic cells and endothelial cells	Marker of hemopoietic stem cells and hematogones. Variable expression in B and T-LBL
CD10	Cell membrane metalloprotease expressed by early B lymphocytes and germinal center B cells. Also known as common acute lymphoblastic leukemia antigen (CALLA)	Positive in most, but not all, cases of B-LBL and in some cases of T-LBL
CD1a	Transmembrane glycoprotein expressed on cortical thymocytes and interdigitating dendritic cells	Positive in some cases of T-LBL (also marks Langerhans cell histiocytosis)
CD99	Glycoprotein normally expressed on thymocytes	Positive in some cases of T-LBL (also marks selected non-hemopoietic neoplasms such as Ewing sarcoma and granulosa cell tumor)
MIB1	Recognizes the Ki67 antigen – a nuclear protein associated with cell proliferation	Generally (but not always) high in LBL (over 60%)
Cyclin D1	Cyclin protein involved in cell cycle regulation, over-expressed in mantle cell lymphoma	Negative staining in LBL is useful in excluding mantle cell lymphoma (in particular the blastoid variant)
CD117	C-kit protein kinase expressed on common myeloid precursor cells	Negative in LBL; useful in excluding myeloid leukemia or myeloid sarcoma
MPO	Myeloperoxidase enzyme found in neutrophil granules	Negative in LBL; positive staining indicates a myeloid leukemia or myeloid sarcoma
CD68	Glycoprotein expressed on monocytes and macrophages	Marker of myeloid or myelo-monocytic cells in myeloid sarcoma. Negative in LBL

Abbreviation: LBL, lymphoblastic leukemia/lymphoma.

- The "lineage infidelity" of LBL alluded to above means that extended immunohistochemistry panels are required. It is advisable to use more than one B lineage and one T lineage marker.

- Beware the effects of treatment. The tumor cells in LBL are extremely sensitive to the effect of steroids given prior to the biopsy. Steroid treatment can alter the cellular morphology in LBL, leading to larger cells with paler nuclei. There may also be a variable effect on immunohistochemistry, with a number of markers being weaker than usual.

- Apparent lymph node involvement by T-LBL external to the mediastinum should raise the possibility of an underlying myeloid neoplasm with an FGFR1 abnormality (8p11 myeloproliferative syndrome).[20] In this rare condition patients may present with chronic eosinophilic leukemia, acute myeloid leukemia, T-LBL or occasionally B-LBL. The leukemia can show a mixed phenotype and may be reported as a bilineal myeloid/T cell lesion. Cytogenetic analysis of bone marrow or lymph node will confirm the diagnosis.

References

1. Lin P, Jones D, Dorfman DM, Medeiros LJ. Precursor B-cell lymphoblastic lymphoma: a predominantly extranodal tumor with low propensity for leukemic involvement. *Am J Surg Pathol* 2000;**24**:1480–1490.

2. Lai R, Hirsch-Ginsberg CF, Bueso-Ramos C. Pathologic diagnosis of acute lymphocytic leukemia. *Hematol Oncol Clin North Am* 2000;**14**:1209–1235.

3. Onciu M. Acute lymphoblastic leukemia. *Hematol Oncol Clin North Am* 2009;**23**:655–674.

4. Portell CA, Sweetenham JW. Adult lymphoblastic lymphoma. *Cancer J* 2012;**18**:432–438.

5. Cortelazzo S, Ponzoni M, Ferreri AJ, Hoelzer D. Lymphoblastic lymphoma. *Crit Rev Oncol Hematol* 2011;**79**:330–343.

6. Faber J, Kantarjian H, Roberts MW, et al. Terminal deoxynucleotidyl transferase-negative acute lymphoblastic leukemia. *Arch Pathol Lab Med* 2000;**124**:92–97.

7. Liu L, McGavran L, Lovell MA, et al. Nonpositive terminal deoxynucleotidyl transferase in pediatric precursor B-lymphoblastic leukemia. *Am J Clin Pathol* 2004;**121**:810–815.

8. Brcić I, Labar B, Perić-Balja M, Basić-Kinda S, Nola M. Terminal deoxynucleotidyl transferase negative T-cell lymphoblastic lymphoma in aleukemic patient. *Int J Hematol* 2008;**88**:189–191.

9. Terada T. TDT⁻, KIT⁺, CD34⁺, CD99⁺ precursor T lymphoblastic leukemia/lymphoma. *Int J Clin Exp Pathol* 2012;**5**:167–170.

10. Al Gwaiz LA, Bassioni W. Immunophenotyping of acute lymphoblastic leukemia using immunohistochemistry in bone marrow biopsy specimens. *Histol Histopathol* 2008;**23**:1223–1228.

11. Feldman AL, Dogan A. Diagnostic uses of Pax5 immunohistochemistry. *Adv Anat Pathol* 2007;**14**:323–334.

12. Pilozzi E, Pulford K, Jones M, et al. Co-expression of CD79a (JCB117) and CD3 by lymphoblastic lymphoma. *J Pathol* 1998;**186**:140–143.

13. Cheng AL, Su IJ, Tien HF, et al. Characteristic clinicopathologic features of adult B-cell lymphoblastic lymphoma with special emphasis on differential diagnosis with an atypical form probably of blastic lymphocytic lymphoma of intermediate differentiation origin. *Cancer* 1994;**73**:706–710.

14. Peterson MR, Noskoviak KJ, Newbury R. CD5-positive B-cell acute lymphoblastic leukemia. *Pediatr Dev Pathol* 2007;**10**:41–45.

15. Cascavilla N, Musto P, D'Arena G, et al. Adult and childhood acute lymphoblastic leukemia: clinico-biological differences based on CD34 antigen expression. *Haematologica* 1997;**82**:31–37.

16. Ozdemirli M, Fanburg-Smith JC, Hartmann DP, Azumi N, Miettinen M. Differentiating lymphoblastic lymphoma and Ewing's sarcoma: lymphocyte markers and gene rearrangement. *Mod Pathol* 2001;**14**:1175–1182.

17. Nowicki M, Miśkowiak B, Kaczmarek-Kanold M. Correlation between early treatment failure and Ki67 antigen expression in blast cells of children with acute lymphoblastic leukaemia before commencing treatment. A retrospective study. *Oncology* 2002;**62**:55–59.

18. Soslow RA, Zukerberg LR, Harris NL, Warnke RA. BCL-1 (PRAD-1/cyclin D-1) overexpression distinguishes the blastoid variant of mantle cell lymphoma from B-lineage lymphoblastic lymphoma. *Mod Pathol* 1997;**10**:810–817.

19. Pai I, Hegde V, Wilson PO, et al. Ectopic thymus presenting as a subglottic mass: diagnostic and management dilemmas. *Int J Pediatr Otorhinolaryngol* 2005;**69**:573–576.

20. Jackson CC, Medeiros LJ, Miranda RN. 8p11 myeloproliferative syndrome: a review. *Hum Pathol* 2010;**41**:461–476.

11 Illustrative case: Lymphoblastic leukemia/lymphoma

Illustrative case

History: Male aged 12. Two week history of dyspnea. Bilateral lymphadenopathy in cervical and subclavicular regions. Mediastinal mass and large right pleural effusion. Clinically suspicious of Hodgkin or non-Hodgkin lymphoma. Biopsy of left cervical lymph node.

Comments: The biopsy shows effacement of the normal nodal architecture by a diffuse sheet of monomorphic small lymphoid cells. At the edge of the biopsy, and focally within the core itself, there are tumor cells that show the effects of traction – the nuclei are ovoid to spindle shaped and aligned in well-defined parallel "streams." At higher power the

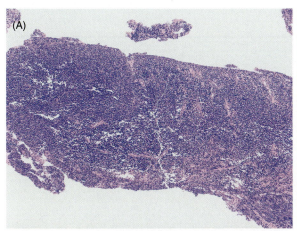

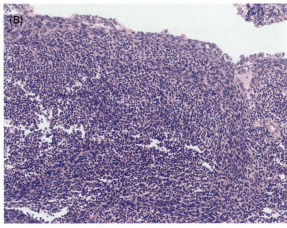

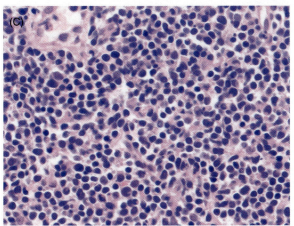

Illustrative case (A–D) H&E sections from this core biopsy show a diffuse infiltrate of monomorphic small to medium-sized lymphoid cells. The cells show focal areas in which the nuclei have been elongated by traction artefact (B). The infiltrating cells have dark irregular nuclei, small nucleoli and little cytoplasm (D). Both CD3 (E) and CD5 (F) are positive and PAX5 (G) is negative. CD20 staining was also negative. The tumor cell nuclei are strongly TdT positive (H) and MIB1 shows a high proliferation fraction (I).

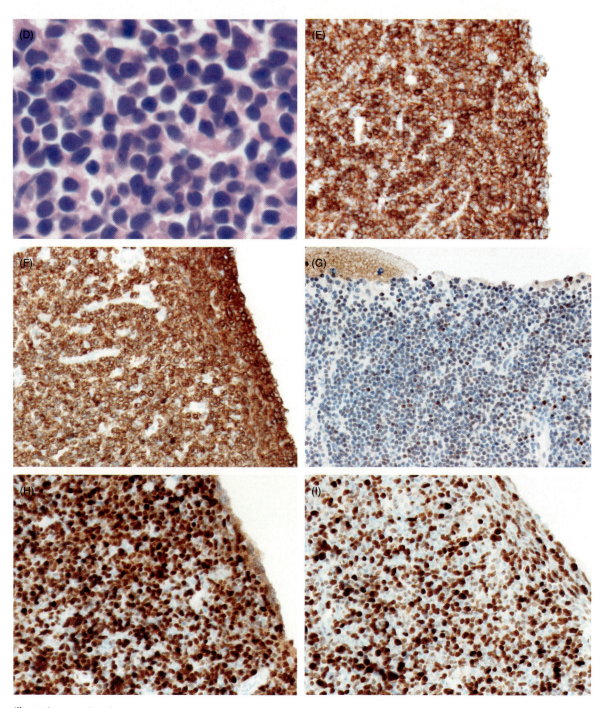

Illustrative case (cont.)

infiltrating cells have dark irregular nuclei with small nucleoli and little cytoplasm. Admixed with the tumor cells are scattered histiocytes, with prominent amounts of eosinophilic cytoplasm. The tumor shows a T cell phenotype, with expression of CD3 and CD5 and negative staining with PAX5 and CD20. TdT shows strong nuclear positivity and MIB1 shows a proliferation fraction of 60–70%.

This case shows the typical features of T lymphoblastic leukemia/lymphoma. A mediastinal mass and pleural effusion are frequent clinical findings. The cellular morphology and phenotype are those of T lymphoblasts. The condition here was at the lymphomatous end of the clinical spectrum – a bone marrow aspirate and trephine biopsy taken shortly after this biopsy showed no evidence of infiltration by leukemia.

Chapter 12

Nodal mature T cell lymphomas

According to the most recent World Health Organization (WHO) classification,[1] peripheral T cell lymphomas (PTCLs) are lymphomas of post-thymic origin and represent approximately 15% of all non-Hodgkin lymphomas in Western populations. The WHO recognizes several clinical subtypes: leukemic/disseminated, nodal and extranodal; the nodal subtype is the most frequent.

Nodal PTCL are clinically and biologically heterogeneous and include: PTCL, not otherwise specified (PTCL-NOS; 25.9% of PTCLs) (Box 12.1); angioimmunoblastic T cell lymphoma (AITL; 18.5%) (Boxes 12.2, 12.3); and anaplastic large cell lymphoma (ALCL). The latter, ALCL, is further separated into ALK positive and ALK negative, accounting for 6.6% and 5.5% of PTCL cases respectively (Boxes 12.4, 12.5).[2] Finally, PTCL-NOS remains a "wastebasket" category, analogous to diffuse large B cell lymphoma, not otherwise specified (DLBCL-NOS), and includes all cases not falling into one of the more specific categories. The morphology and the immunophenotype are complex with frequent aberrant T cell phenotypes (Tables 12.1, 12.2[3]).

Among the disseminated forms, adult T cell leukemia/lymphoma (ATLL), presents with widespread nodal involvement and will be briefly discussed in this chapter (Box 12.6). Some extranodal lymphomas such as extranodal NK/T cell lymphoma, nasal type and enteropathy-associated T cell lymphoma (EATL) may show secondary lymph node involvement but are very rarely seen in lymph node core biopsies.

Differential diagnosis

The differential diagnosis of nodal PTCL includes other B and T cell lymphomas and, most importantly, non-neoplastic lesions in which clinicopathological correlation is paramount (serology, clinically indolent, isolated lymphadenopathy, spontaneous resolution, etc.).

Non-neoplastic (see also Chapters 1 and 2)

1. Kikuchi lymphadenitis (KL; Kikuchi–Fujimoto disease). Sheets of atypical T cells/immunoblasts can be seen but these are usually CD8 positive,

---

Box 12.1 Peripheral T cell lymphoma, not otherwise specified (PTCL-NOS)

Morphology	Paracortical or diffuse neoplastic population with broad cytological spectrum from medium-sized to large cells with pleomorphic nuclei (Fig. 12.1A,B), Reed–Sternberg-like cells and clear cells are also present. T cell pattern not specific. Some cases show increased high endothelial venules. Background mixed with small lymphocytes, epithelioid histiocytes, eosinophils and occasionally large B cells
Immunophenotype	• Aberrant T cell immunophenotype in 70% of cases (downregulation of CD5 and CD7), T cell receptor beta-chain antibody BF1 usually expressed. Aberrant expression of B cell markers is seen in some cases
	• Variable expression of CD30[4] and positivity with T_{FH} cell markers (ICOS, PD1 and CXCL13 – Fig. 12.1C; CXCL13 and ICOS – Fig. 12.1D). CD30-positive and CD30-negative forms of PTCL-NOS may represent two biological diseases with different clinical outcomes[5]
	• High-proliferation fraction (±70%) (Fig. 12.1E)

Follicular variant   Intrafollicular aggregates of atypical T cells, usually with clear cell morphology or "perifollicular" aggregates of T cells mimicking marginal zone lymphoma. Lack high endothelial venules or follicular dendritic cell expanded meshworks, but share T_{FH} phenotype with AITL[6]

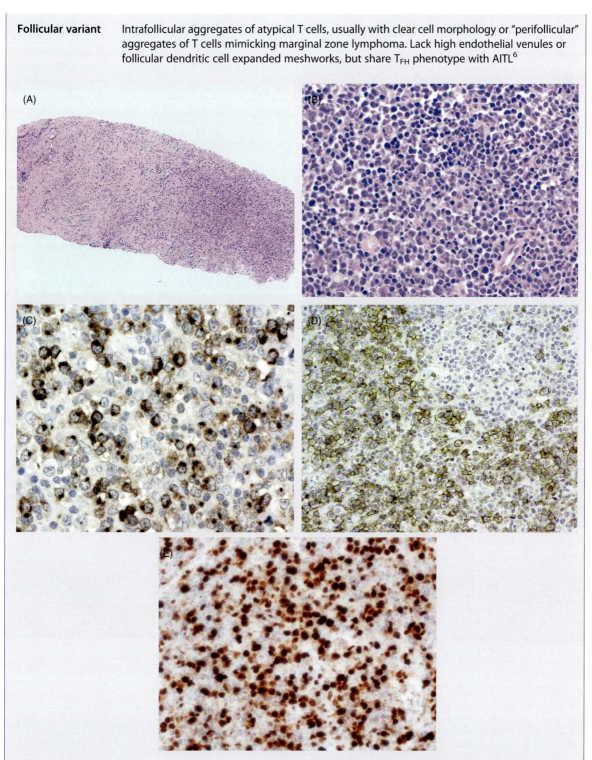

Figure 12.1 **Peripheral T cell lymphoma, not otherwise specified (PTCL-NOS).** Core biopsy showing diffuse effacement of the normal architecture; at low power eosinophils and a mixed lymphoid population are noted (A, H&E). In some cases the neoplastic population is very pleomorphic with large cells resembling Hodgkin Reed–Sternberg (HRS) cells (B, H&E). Expression of T_{FH} cell markers can be seen in cases of PTCL-NOS (C is CXL13 and D is ICOS). The proliferation fraction with MIB-1 in PTCL is usually high (E).

Box 12.2 Angioimmunoblastic T cell lymphoma (AITL)

Morphology	Partial or diffuse effacement of the nodal architecture by a paracortical expansion of small to medium-sized lymphocytes, some with clear cytoplasm and marked proliferation of high endothelial venules (Fig. 12.2A–C). Regressed or absent follicles. Expansion of follicular dendritic cells around high endothelial venules (Fig. 12.2D – CD21 stain). Frequent presence of clusters of neoplastic cells around high endothelial venules and residual follicles. Polymorphic background population including plasma cells, epithelioid histiocytes and eosinophils
Immunophenotype	• Positive with pan-T cell markers (CD2, CD3, CD5), normally CD4 positive but numerous CD8 positive reactive T cells also present
	• Classical T_{FH} immunophenotype: bcl-6, CD10, CXCL13 and PD1 positivity in 60–100% [7] (Fig. 12.3A)
	• EBV-positive, CD20-positive large cells (CD20 – Fig. 12.3B; EBER – Fig. 12.3C)
	• 90% TCR clonally rearranged, 10–20% IgG clonally rearranged

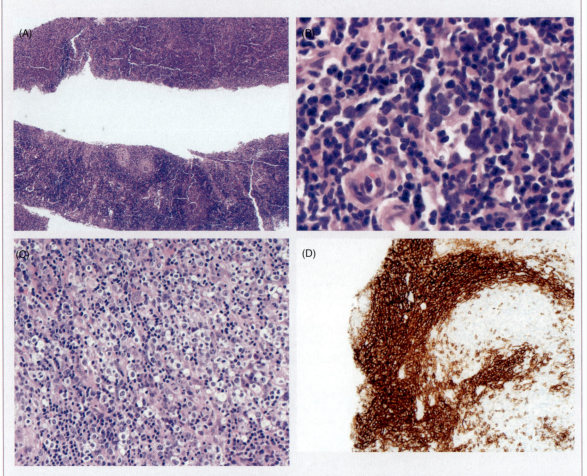

Figure 12.2 Angioimmunoblastic T cell lymphoma (AITL). Core biopsies showing effacement of the normal architecture by a diffuse infiltrate with a prominent vascular pattern (A, H&E). There is wide variation in the morphology of tumor cells, some cases contain large cells in a background of small lymphocytes (B) and in some cases clusters of clear cells (C) are found. Proliferation of follicular dendritic cell (FDC) meshworks encircling vessels are best highlighted with CD21 (D).

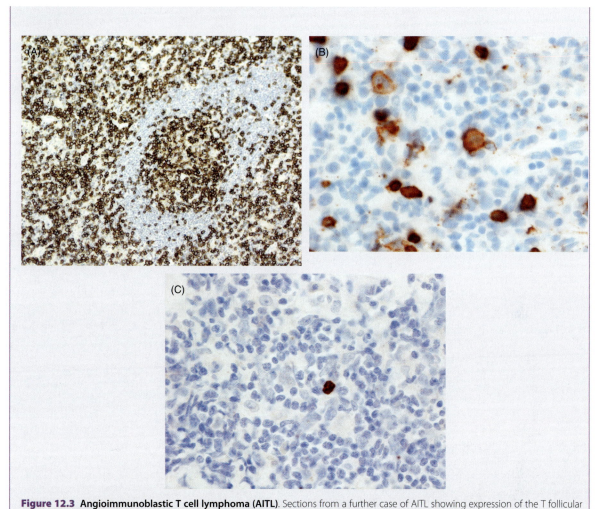

Figure 12.3 Angioimmunoblastic T cell lymphoma (AITL). Sections from a further case of AITL showing expression of the T follicular helper marker PD1 (A). PD1 is positive in 60–100% of AITL cases; note that the staining intensity of the neoplastic T cells outside the follicle is as strong as that of the normal follicular T cells within the germinal center. Almost invariably all cases of AITL contain large CD20 positive B cells (B) that are usually EBV positive (C, EBER in-situ hybridization).

show no aberrant T cell phenotype and are polyclonal. Foci of non-suppurative necrosis are almost always present in KL but necrosis is rare in PTCL. Histiocytes can be present in both conditions but in KL they show typical crescentic morphology and show cytoplasmic expression of MPO.

2. Granulomatous lymphadenitis. Clusters of epithelioid histiocytes and a background rich in small lymphocytes can be found in PTCL but reactive granulomatous lymphadenitis lacks cytological atypia, the lymph node architecture is

preserved and the T cells show no loss of pan-T cell markers.

3. Dermatopathic lymphadenopathy. Regressed follicles, paracortical expansion of histiocytes, plasma cells, eosinophils and a prominent vascular pattern can be seen in both PTCL and dermatopathic lymphadenopathy. The presence of pale staining, interdigitating dendritic cells (S100 positive and CD1a positive) and pigment laden macrophages favors a diagnosis of dermatopathic lymphadenopathy. However, cases of dermatopathic lymphadenopathy can have

Box 12.3 Anaplastic large cell lymphoma (ALCL), ALK positive

Morphology	Variable presence of hallmark cells with eccentric, horseshoe or kidney-shaped nuclei identified in almost all cases (Fig. 12.4A,B). Several patterns: (i) "common" with classical large cells and some cells resembling Reed–Sternberg cells; (ii) lymphohistiocytic in which the neoplastic cells can be difficult to identify due to the striking histiocytic component, (iii) small cell variant; and (iv) rare variants – sarcomatoid, signet-ring cell and neutrophil-rich. An intrasinusoidal pattern of infiltration is characteristic[8]
Immunophenotype	• CD30 positive in cell membrane and Golgi region (Fig. 12.4C)
	• ALK shows both nuclear and cytoplasmic positive staining (Fig. 12.4D) and the distribution may reflect variant translocations[9]
	• T cell lineage markers are positive, most frequently CD2, but cases can show loss of one or several pan-T antigens. Some cases are of "null-cell type" and do not express T lineage markers, but there is evidence of T cell lineage using molecular studies. Positivity for cytotoxic markers: TIA1, granzyme B and/or perforin. Rarely CD15 positive. EBER consistently negative

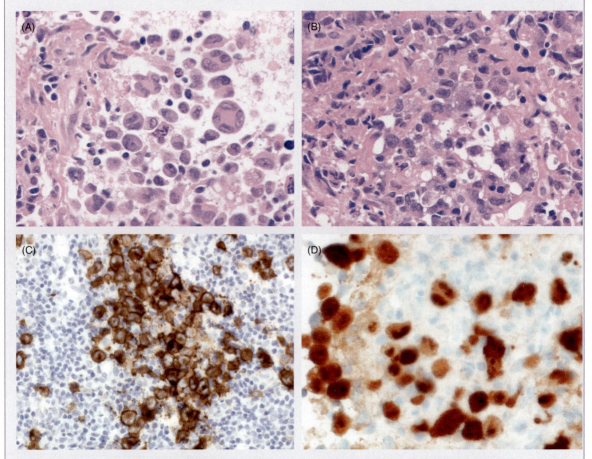

Figure 12.4 Anaplastic large cell lymphoma (ALCL), ALK positive. In addition to hallmark cells, cases of ALCL also show multinucleated giant cells and HRS-like cells mimicking classical Hodgkin lymphoma (CHL) (A,B). CD30 immunostaining is usually strong and highlights intra-sinusoidal tumor cell aggregates (C). ALK1 is positive in both the nucleus and cytoplasm (D).

Box 12.4 Anaplastic large cell lymphoma (ALCL), ALK negative[10]

Morphology	Effacement of architecture by sheets of neoplastic cells larger and more pleomorphic than ALCL, ALK positive (Fig. 12.5A,B). The neoplastic cells are pleomorphic, some multinucleated, with prominent nucleoli. Hallmark cells and intrasinusoidal involvement are also seen. Some cases can show sclerosis and numerous eosinophils
Immunophenotype	CD30 membrane and Golgi positivity, strong and diffuse. Loss of some pan-T cell markers, CD4 commonly positive and CD8 rarely positive. Cytotoxic markers usually positive. EMA rarely expressed (Fig. 12.5C). EBER negative and EBV-LMP1 negative

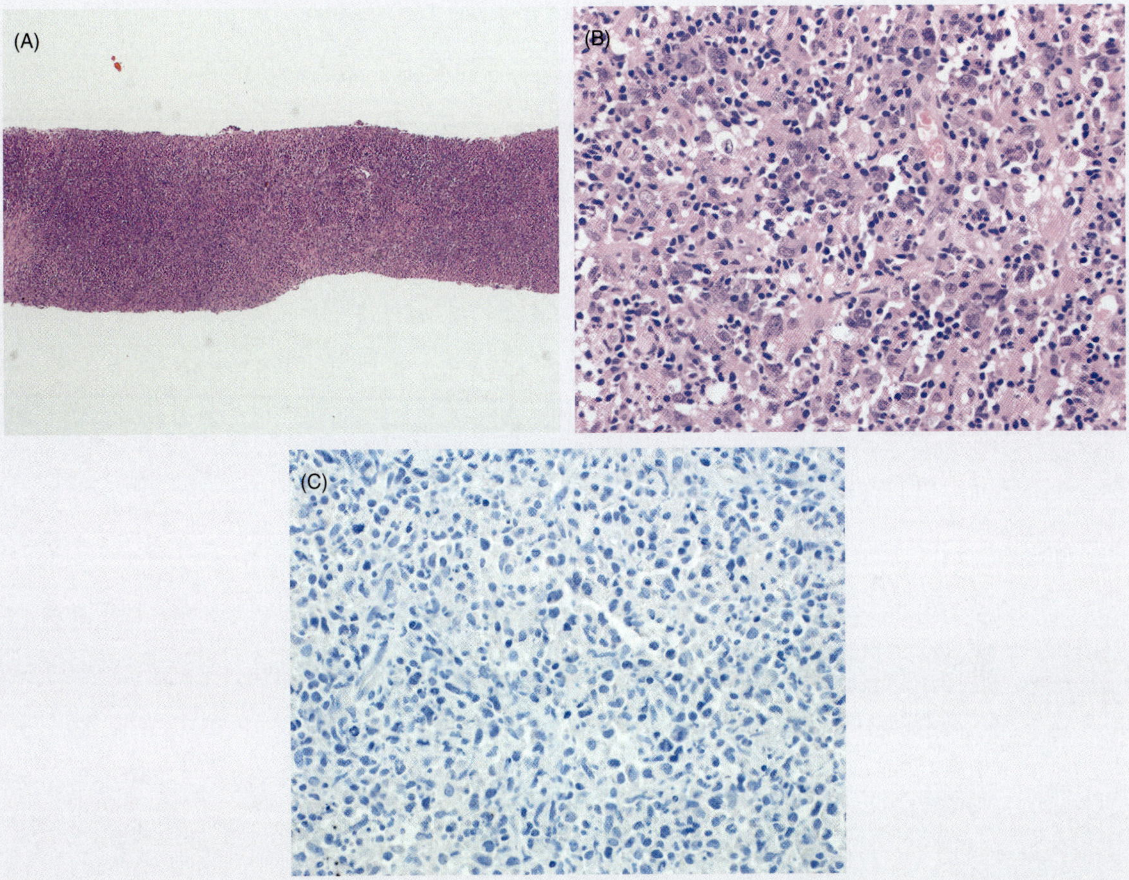

Figure 12.5 Anaplastic large cell lymphoma (ALCL), ALK negative. Core biopsy showing effacement of the normal architecture by a diffuse infiltrate composed of sheets of atypical lymphoid cells (A, H&E). The cells are larger and more pleomorphic than those seen in ALCL, ALK positive; some are multinucleated and many have prominent nucleoli (B, H&E). Unlike ALCL, ALK positive, EMA staining is usually negative (C).

concomitant involvement by cutaneous T cell lymphoma with cytologically malignant T cells. The latter often show an aberrant T cell immunophenotype and polymerase chain reaction (PCR) will show a T cell clonal expansion.

4. Viral infections. Immunoblasts in expanded paracortical zones, prominent vessels and Reed–Sternberg-like cells are noted in reactive viral lymphadenitis and in PTCL. Reed–Sternberg-like cells are usually of T cell lineage in viral infections and have a B cell origin in PTCL. Similarly Epstein–Barr virus (EBV)-positive cells are commonly B cells in PTCL and T cells in viral infections such as infectious mononucleosis.

Box 12.5 Adult T cell leukemia/lymphoma (ATLL)

Morphology	Mainly highly pleomorphic lymphoid cells but a small cell variant (small lymphocytes with irregular nuclear contours), an anaplastic variant and cases resembling AITL exist. (Fig. 12.6A,B) In early phases it can mimic classical Hodgkin lymphoma with a paracortical expansion containing a diffuse infiltrate of small/medium pleomorphic cells and Reed–Sternberg-like cells.[11] There can also be eosinophilia
Immunophenotype	• CD2 positive, CD3 positive and CD5 positive, but CD7 normally negative. Usually CD4 positive and CD8 negative • Large transformed cells (Reed–Sternberg-like cells) are both CD30 and EBER positive but ALK/cytotoxic markers negative • Usually regulatory immunophenotype: both FOXP3 and CCR4 positive • CD25 positive (Fig. 12.6C) in almost 100% of cases.[12] Some cases can also be positive with myeloid markers (CD13 and CD33, Fig. 12.6D)

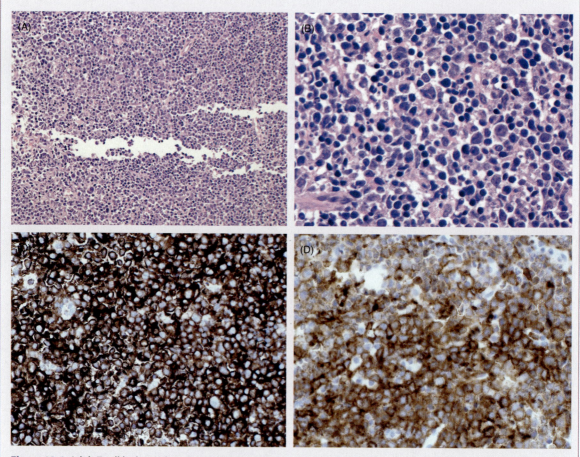

Figure 12.6 Adult T cell leukemia/lymphoma (ATLL). Core biopsy showing a sheet of medium-sized to large mononuclear pleomorphic lymphoid cells with prominent nucleoli (A,B). CD25 is diffusely positive in the majority of cases (C) but expression of CD33 has also been described, and can lead to possible diagnostic confusion with a myeloid neoplasm (D).

Table 12.1 Immunohistochemical panel for investigation of T cell lymphoma

Antibody	Specificity	Utility
CD3	Pan-T cell marker – part of the protein complex associated with the T cell receptor	Stains the majority of T cell lymphomas. ALCL can be CD3 negative
CD5	T cell surface glycoprotein, pan-T cell marker	Positive in some ATLL, AITL and some PTCL-NOS. Negative in ALCL
CD4	T cell helper population	Positive in the majority of nodal PTCL. Can be positive in some cases of AML with monocytic differentiation
CD8	T cell cytotoxic population	Usually negative in mature T cell neoplasms but positive in some PTCL-NOS and EATL cases
CD2	Pan-T cell marker, thymocytes and NK cells	Preserved expression in the majority of mature T cell neoplasms, including both ALCL, ALK positive and ALCL, ALK negative
CD7	Pan-T cell marker. Myeloid and NK cells can also be positive	Expression usually lost in ALCL, ATLL, EATL and some cases of PTCL-NOS
CD30	Cell membrane protein in the tumor necrosis factor receptor family; marks activated lymphoid cells	Positive in ALCL but also expressed in some cases of PTCL-NOS, EATL and ATLL
CD56	NK-cell marker and a subset of T cells and myeloid cells	Subset of PTCL-NOS, ALCL, ALK positive. EATL can be positive
ALK1	Anaplastic lymphoma kinase; tyrosine kinase receptor	Over-expressed in ALCL, ALK positive
CXCL13	C-X-C motif chemokine 13 (CXCL13) also known as B lymphocyte chemoattractant	T follicular helper cell marker. Sensitive marker for AITL but also expressed in non-AITL mature T cell lymphomas
ICOS	Inducible T cell co-stimulator, expressed in activated T cells	T follicular helper cell marker. Sensitive marker for AITL and PTCL-follicular variant, but up to 50% of PTCL-NOS can be positive
PD1	Also known as Programmed cell death protein 1 or CD279, member of the CD28/CTLA-4 T cell regulators	T follicular helper cell marker. Sensitive marker for AITL (highest sensitivity but lower specificity) but also expressed in non-AITL mature T cell lymphomas and, rarely, in B cell lymphomas
EBER	Epstein–Barr encoded viral RNA	NK lymphomas and B cells in PTCL and AITL
CD10	Common ALL antigen positive in germinal center B cells and B cell precursors	Positive in T-LBL, a subset of PTCL-NOS and up to 50% of AITL. In AITL CD10 has the highest specificity but lowest sensitivity
BCL-6	Transcription factor expressed in the nuclei of germinal center B cells	Positive in PTCL-NOS and AITL
TdT	Terminal deoxynucleotidyl transferase	Expressed in precursor T cells, B cells and LBL. Merkel cell carcinoma and some lung small cell carcinomas can also be positive
CD103	Intraepithelial/mucosal T cells	Positive in EATL but also in some cases of ATLL and in hairy cell leukemia
TIA-1	T cell-restricted intracellular antigen 1	Expressed in EATL and in some cases of ALCL (both ALK positive and ALK negative) and PTCL-NOS
Granzyme B	Cytotoxic T cell marker	Expressed in EATL and in some cases of ALCL (both ALK positive and ALK negative) and PTCL-NOS
Perforin	Cytotoxic T cell marker	Expressed in EATL and in some cases of ALCL (both ALK positive and ALK negative) and PTCL-NOS
CD13	Myeloid marker	Some ALCL cases can express this myeloid marker
CD33	Myeloid marker	Positive staining in some cases of ALCL
CD52	Reacts with the human CD52 antigen, also known as CAMPATH-1	High expression in PTCL-NOS and AITL. Low expression in ALCL
CD20	Transmembrane protein expressed early in B cell development	Expression of CD20 and/or CD79a has been described in rare cases of PTCL-NOS

Abbreviations: AITL, angioimmunoblastic T cell lymphoma; ALCL, anaplastic large cell lymphoma; ALL, acute lymphoblastic leukemia; AML, acute myeloid leukemia; ATLL, adult T cell leukemia/lymphoma; EATL, enteropathy-associated T cell lymphoma; PTCL-NOS, peripheral T cell lymphoma, not otherwise specified; T-LBL, T cell lymphoblastic leukemia/lymphoma.

Table 12.2 Immunophenotype of PTCL

	PTCL-NOS	AITL	ATLL	T-LBL	ALCL, ALK positive	ALCL, ALK negative	EATL	NK
Myeloid markers	Negative (–)	–	–	CD13 and CD33 positive in some cases	–	–	–	–
B cell markers	Positive in bystander B cells and a variable fraction of tumor cells	EBV+ CD20+ large B cells present in most cases	–	CD79a positive in some cases	–	–	–	–
TdT	–	–	–	+	–	–	–	–
CD30	+/–	–/+	+/–	–	+	+	+	–/+
Cytotoxic	–	–	–	–	+	+	+	+/–
CD4	Variable. CD4 positivity is commoner than CD8 positivity	Tumor cells positive in most cases	+	–	+	+	–	–
CD8	–/+ *	Positive in background reactive CD8 T cells	–/+	–	–/+	–/+	–/+	–
CD56	–/+	–	–	–	–	–	+ (EATL type II)	+
EBER/LMP1	Positive in B immunoblasts in lymphoepitheliod variant	Positive in CD20+ large B cells	–	–	–	–	–	+
ALK	–	–	–	–	+	–	–	–
T$_{FH}$	–/+ †	+	–	–	–	–	–	–
Others	CD52–/+	CD10+/– Bcl-6+/–	FoxP3+/– CD25+ CD15–/+	CD1a+/– CD10+/– CD99+/–	EMA +ve	EMA–/+ Clusterin+	CD103+	

Abbreviations: AITL, angioimmunoblastic T cell lymphoma; ALCL, anaplastic large cell lymphoma; ATLL, adult T cell leukemia/lymphoma; EATL, enteropathy-associated T cell lymphoma; EBV, Epstein–Barr virus; NK, extranodal NK/T cell lymphoma nasal type; PTCL-NOS, peripheral T cell lymphoma, not otherwise specified; T-LBL, T lymphoblastic lymphoma (see Chapter 11).
Cytotoxic markers: TIA-1, Granzyme B and perforin.
T$_{FH}$ cell markers: PD1, CXCL13 and ICOS.
* The majority of neoplastic cells are CD8 positive in the lymphoepithelioid variant.[3]
† Positive in almost all cases of follicular variant of PTCL-NOS.

5. Reactive T zone (paracortical) hyperplasia. In contrast with PTCL the architecture is usually preserved, the T cell population lacks significant cytological atypia and comprises a mixed population of both CD4 and CD8-positive T cells. However, variable expression of CD25 and CD30 and, occasionally, CD20-positive B cells can also be present in reactive T zone hyperplasia.

Neoplastic (see also Chapters 3 and 9)

- Classical Hodgkin lymphoma and PTCL can both show large CD30-positive, EBV-positive and CD20-positive Reed–Sternberg-like cells and a polymorphic background containing eosinophils and epithelioid histiocytes. The presence of paracortical expansion with preservation of germinal centers and an atypical population of T cells (with or without aberrant phenotype) can assist in the differential diagnosis. Some cases of ALCL, ALK positive can mimic nodular sclerosis classical Hodgkin lymphoma (NS-CHL) and it has been suggested that ALK staining should be performed in cases with morphological features of NS-CHL that are EMA positive and CD15 negative.[13] ALCL, ALK negative cases were previously classified as "Hodgkin-like" ALCL.

- T cell/histiocyte-rich large B cell lymphoma usually contains a small number of large neoplastic B cells (less than 10% of lymphoid population) in a background rich in T cells, often with accompanying epithelioid histiocytes. In PTCL the T cell population is cytologically malignant and, as mentioned before, can show aberrant loss of pan-T cell markers. Although the T cells are usually monoclonal, immunoglobulin gene rearrangement can be seen in up to 30% of PTCL, making the diagnosis very challenging.

- DLBCL and ALCL, ALK positive, particularly in cases with immunoblastic morphology and prominent sinusoidal growth pattern. In ALK-positive large B cell lymphoma, although the neoplastic cells can be EMA positive, there is absence of CD30, a paucity of normal B and T lineage markers and strong expression of CD138 and/or VS38c. ALK is usually granular and confined to the cytoplasm with very rare or absent nuclear staining.

- The differential diagnosis of PTCL with AITL and ALCL is discussed in the following section.

Peripheral T cell lymphoma: problems and pitfalls of core biopsies

- ALCL small cell variant (5–10% of ALCL) is composed of a population of small to medium-size cells with irregular nuclei and pale cytoplasm. The possibility of PTCL-NOS should be considered in these cases. Although scanty, hallmark cells around blood vessels along with negativity of neoplastic cells with CD3 favor the small cell variant of ALCL.

- EBV-positive B cells have been reported in AITL and other PTCLs and may mimic Hodgkin/Reed–Sternberg (HRS) cells. EBV negative HRS-like B cells may also occur in the background of PTCL; caution is needed to avoid misdiagnosis as CHL.[14] Rarely the large cells may also express CD30 and CD15. Although weak PAX5 staining favors CHL, rare cases of ALCL may be weakly positive with PAX5.[15]

- ALCL, lymphohistiocytic variant can be mistaken for an infective or reactive process and, where there is strong clinical suspicion of lymphoma, repeat biopsy may be necessary.

- A subset of PTCL-NOS are strongly CD30 positive, can co-express CD15 and can morphologically resemble ALCL, ALK negative.[16]

- T cells in PTCL are normally monoclonal or oligoclonal but monoclonal immunoglobulin gene rearrangement can be found in up to one-third of cases. In addition aberrant expression of CD20 and CD79a can also occur in PTCL-NOS.[17]

- PD1 expression can be seen in both AITL and in reactive paracortical hyperplasia but the intensity of the staining can help in the differential diagnosis. In reactive paracortical hyperplasia, the small T cells are usually PD1 weakly positive in comparison with strong staining in the T cells within the germinal centers. In summary, only strong PD1 expression is useful in the diagnosis of AITL (Fig. 12.3A).

- Although TdT and CD99 are consistently expressed in T cell lymphoblastic leukemia/lymphoma (T-LBL), non-lymphoid tumors with a similar morphology can also express TdT (e.g. Merkel cell carcinoma and small cell carcinoma of the lung[18]). Expression of CD99 has also been reported in ALCL, ALK positive cases.[19]

- AITL with hyperplastic germinal centers (pattern 1) represents a difficult diagnosis. It is frequently misdiagnosed as reactive hyperplasia as this pattern lacks prominent accumulation of follicular dendritic cells encircling high endothelial venules and the neoplastic population can be scanty. Aggregates of atypical PD1 positive cells around the follicles (perifollicular pattern in the outer zone of the follicle) and the presence of atypical EBV-positive B cells favor a diagnosis of AITL.[20]

- The follicular variant of PTCL-NOS shares some morphological and immunohistochemical features with AITL and there can be an overlap between these two entities. In PTCL follicular variant the neoplastic cells are confined to the follicle, lack CD10 expression and there is no significant expansion of follicular dendritic cell meshworks outside the follicles.[6]

References

1. Swerdlow S, Campo E, Harris N, et al. *WHO Classification of Tumours of Haematopoietic and Lymphoid Tissues*, 4th edn. Lyon, France: International Agency for Research on Cancer; 2008.

2. Foss FM, Zinzani PL, Vose JM, et al. Peripheral T-cell lymphoma. *Blood* 2011;**117**:6756–6767.

3. Geissinger E, Odenwald T, Lee SS, et al. Nodal peripheral T-cell lymphomas and, in particular, their lymphoepithelioid (Lennert's) variant are often derived from CD8⁺ cytotoxic T-cells. *Virchows Arch* 2004;**445**:334–343.

4. Kanavaros P, Boulland ML, Petit B, Arnulf B, Gaulard P. Expression of cytotoxic proteins in peripheral T-cell and natural killer-cell (NK) lymphomas: association with extranodal site, NK or T gamma delta phenotype, anaplastic morphology and CD30 expression. *Leuk Lymphoma* 2000;**38**:317–326.

5. Bisig B, de Reyniès A, Bonnet C, et al. Molecular and phenotypic features are shared by CD30-positive peripheral T-cell lymphomas. *Haematologica* 2013;**98**:1250–1258.

6. Rodríguez-Pinilla SM, Atienza L, Murillo C, et al. Peripheral T-cell lymphoma with follicular T-cell markers. *Am J Surg Pathol* 2008;**32**:1787–1799.

7. Roncador G, García Verdes-Montenegro JF, Tedoldi S, et al. Expression of two markers of germinal center T cells (SAP and PD-1) in angioimmunoblastic T-cell lymphoma. *Haematologica* 2007;**92**:1059–1066.

8. Stein H, Foss HD, Dürkop H, et al. CD30⁺ anaplastic large cell lymphoma: a review of its histopathologic, genetic, and clinical features. *Blood* 2000;**96**:3681–3695.

9. Pulford K, Morris SW, Mason DY. Anaplastic lymphoma kinase proteins and malignancy. *Curr Opin Hematol* 2001;**8**:231–236.

10. Savage KJ, Harris NL, Vose JM, et al. ALK⁻ anaplastic large-cell lymphoma is clinically and immunophenotypically different from both ALK⁺ ALCL and peripheral T-cell lymphoma, not otherwise specified: report from the International Peripheral T-cell Lymphoma Project. *Blood* 2008;**111**:5496–5504.

11. Venkataraman G, Berkowitz J, Morris JC, et al. Adult T-cell leukemia/lymphoma with Epstein–Barr virus-positive Hodgkin-like cells. *Hum Pathol* 2011;**42**:1042–1046.

12. Abe M, Uchihashi K, Kazuto T, et al. Foxp3 expression on normal and leukemic CD4⁺CD25⁺ T cells implicated in human T-cell leukemia virus type-1 is inconsistent with Treg cells. *Eur J Haematol* 2008;**81**:209–217.

13. Vassallo J, Lamant L, Brugieres L, et al. ALK-positive anaplastic large cell lymphoma mimicking nodular sclerosis Hodgkin's lymphoma: report of 10 cases. *Am J Surg Pathol* 2006;**30**:223–229.

14. Nicolae A, Pittaluga S, Venkataraman G, et al. Peripheral T-cell lymphomas of follicular T-helper cell derivation with Hodgkin/Reed–Sternberg cells of B-cell lineage: both EBV-positive and EBV-negative variants exist. *Am J Surg Pathol* 2013;**37**:816–826.

15. Feldman AL, Law ME, Inwards DJ, et al. PAX5-positive T-cell anaplastic large cell lymphomas associated with extra copies of the PAX5 gene locus. *Mod Pathol* 2010;**23**:593–602.

16. Barry TS, Jaffe ES, Sorbara L, Raffeld M, Pittaluga S. Peripheral T-cell lymphomas expressing CD30 and CD15. *Am J Surg Pathol* 2003;**27**:1513–1522.

17. Yao X, Teruya-Feldstein J, Raffeld M, Sorbara L, Jaffe ES. Peripheral T-cell lymphoma with aberrant expression of CD79a and CD20: a diagnostic pitfall. *Mod Pathol* 2001;**14**:105–110.

18. Kolhe R, Reid MD, Lee JR, et al. Immunohistochemical expression of PAX5 and TdT by Merkel cell carcinoma and pulmonary small cell carcinoma: a potential diagnostic pitfall but useful discriminatory marker. *Int J Clin Exp Pathol* 2013;**6**:142–147.

19. Buxton D, Bacchi CE, Gualco G, et al. Frequent expression of CD99 in anaplastic large cell lymphoma: a clinicopathologic and immunohistochemical study of 160 cases. *Am J Clin Pathol* 2009;**131**:574–579.

20. Rodriguez-Justo M, Attygalle AD, Munson P, et al. Angioimmunoblastic T-cell lymphoma with hyperplastic germinal centres: a neoplasia with origin in the outer zone of the germinal centre? Clinicopathological and immunohistochemical study of 10 cases with follicular T-cell markers. *Mod Pathol* 2009;**22**:753–761.

12

Illustrative case: Nodal mature T cell lymphomas

Illustrative case

History: Female aged 21 with a 5 year history of chronic phase of chronic myeloid leukemia (CML) on Imatinib, alpha-interferon and intermittent leukophoresis. Presented with a 4 week history of cervical lymphadenopathy. An ultrasound examination suggested that this was abnormal and a computed tomography (CT) guided biopsy was performed.

Comments: This case illustrates T lymphoblastic transformation in a patient with known CML, which is extremely rare, although the possibility of two unrelated diseases should also be considered here. The co-expression of CD79a is reported in 10% of cases of T lymphoblastic leukemia/lymphoma and the clinical implication of this finding is of uncertain significance. CD79a can be expressed in both mature and immature T cell lymphoproliferative disorders.

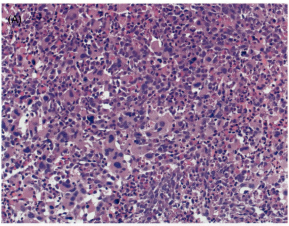

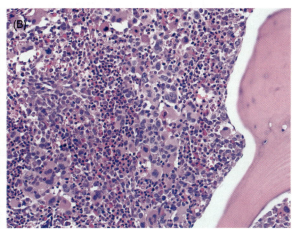

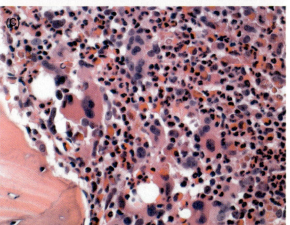

Illustrative case (A–E) Images taken from the bone marrow trephine biopsy. These show a markedly hypercellular marrow with granulocytic and megakaryocytic hyperplasia. Neutrophils and eosinophils are increased. Clusters of megakaryocytes and abnormal forms are seen (A–C). Reticulin is increased (D) and clusters of megakaryocytes are highlighted with CD61 (E).

(F–L) Images from the lymph node. H&E sections (F–H) show effacement of the normal architecture by a relatively monomorphic population of small to medium-sized lymphoid cells with dark irregular nucleoli anad scanty cytoplasm. Immunophenotypically the tumor cells are CD3 positive (I), CD79a positive (J), CD99 positive (K) and show strong nuclear staining with TdT (L).

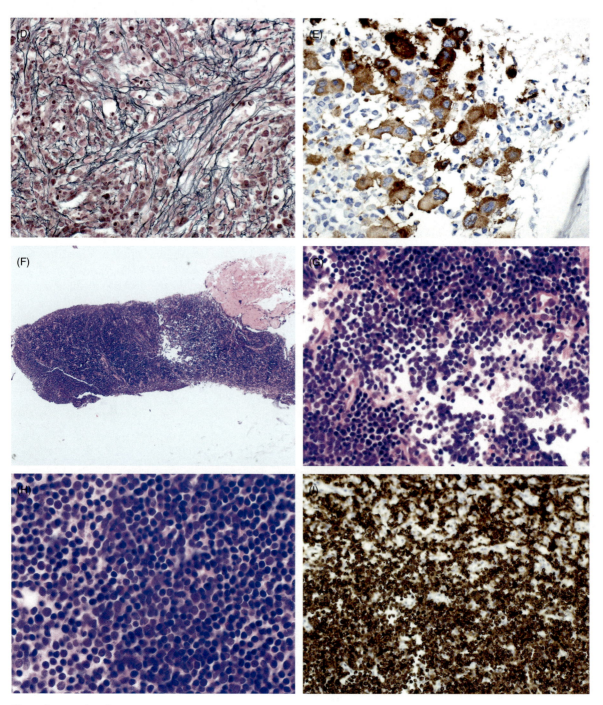

Illustrative case (cont.)

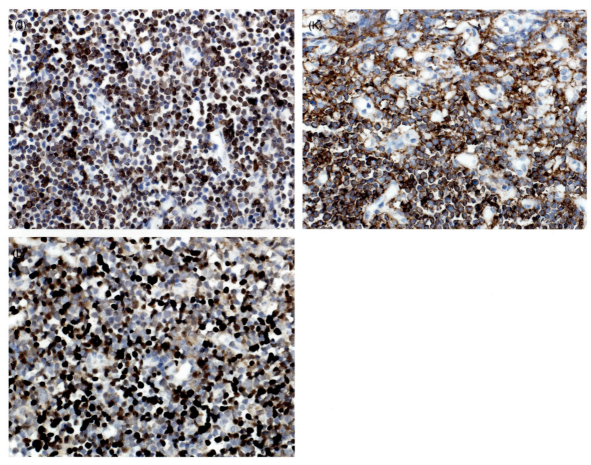

Illustrative case (cont.)

Chapter 13

Plasma cell neoplasms

Plasma cell neoplasms (PCNs) in needle core biopsies may represent extramedullary plasmacytoma, rare examples of plasma cell myeloma spreading outside the bone marrow or plasmablastic lymphoma.[1–3] Plasmacytoma and plasma cell myeloma usually show diffuse sheets of cells with recognizable (mature) plasma cell morphology (Fig. 13.1A–E). The typical plasma cell is oval in outline with eosinophilic or slightly basophilic cytoplasm and an eccentrically placed round nucleus with a "cartwheel" or "clock-face" chromatin pattern, although this is often less marked in PCNs. There may be an area of clearing within the cytoplasm (the "hof") associated with the Golgi apparatus (Fig. 13.1D,E). Atypical and binucleate forms are frequently seen in these neoplasms (Fig. 13.1E). Less well-differentiated examples will include more plasmablastic forms in which the nucleus is more central and the clock-face chromatin is replaced by a single central nucleolus. Amyloid deposition may be seen in association with these lesions. Plasmablastic lymphoma is a high grade B cell neoplasm composed of cells with immunoblastic morphology; there is morphological overlap with diffuse large B cell lymphoma (see Chapter 9).[4,5] There is an association with immunodeficiency and many cases are Epstein–Barr virus (EBV)-associated; the best-known example is the oral plasmablastic lymphoma seen in patients with human immunodeficiency virus (HIV).[6,7]

Immunohistochemistry

Plasma cell neoplasms show a complex immunohistochemical picture (Table 13.1). Mature plasma cells are positive with CD138, CD38, VS38c and MUM1/IRF4 (Fig. 13.1F–I).[8–10] CD45 is often negative but may be positive in plasmablastic lymphoma. B lineage markers show a variable picture: CD79a is positive in many, but not all, cases of PCN; PAX5 is usually negative; CD20 is typically negative (Fig. 13.1G) but can be aberrantly expressed; and both CD19 and CD22 are normally negative.[11,12] In addition the neoplastic plasma cells can stain with a number of "aberrant"

markers not usually seen in mature B cells. These include CD56, CD117, CD33 and cyclin D1 (some PCNs have the t(11;14) CCND1 translocation).[13–17] The cyclin D1-positive PCN cases will often co-express CD20. The neoplastic plasma cells can express EMA and plasmablastic lymphoma can be CD30 positive. CD10 is usually negative (some cases are positive) and bcl-6 can show weak staining; bcl-2 is strongly positive. T cell markers are negative (Fig. 13.1G), but occasional cases can show cytoplasmic expression of CD3, CD2 or CD4.[18] Expression of cytokeratins by neoplastic plasma cells is also recorded.[19] The definitive diagnosis of PCN relies on the detection of light chain restriction (Fig. 13.1I,J). Staining for immunoglobulin light or heavy chains should be cytoplasmic rather than membrane. Polymerase chain reaction (PCR) may be helpful in confirming the clonal nature of a plasma cell infiltrate.

Differential diagnosis

1. Reactive plasma cells. There may be no morphological features that allow the distinction of tumors of mature plasma cells from a reactive plasma cell infiltrate. Binucleate forms are found in both reactive and neoplastic settings. Immunoglobulin light chain staining should show a polytypic picture in reactive conditions and should demonstrate monotypic restriction in PCN. Expression of an aberrant marker such as CD56 or cyclin D1 will also indicate a neoplastic population. PCR may be required to assess clonality.

2. Marginal zone lymphoma (MZL) and lymphoplasmacytic lymphoma (LPL) with plasma cell differentiation may closely resemble PCNs (see Chapter 8).[20] The presence of a CD20-positive, CD138-negative neoplastic population of small lymphocytes will exclude PCN, and the aberrant markers of neoplastic plasma cells are negative in MZL and LPL. IgM is rarely positive in PCNs, but is commonly positive in MZL and LPL.

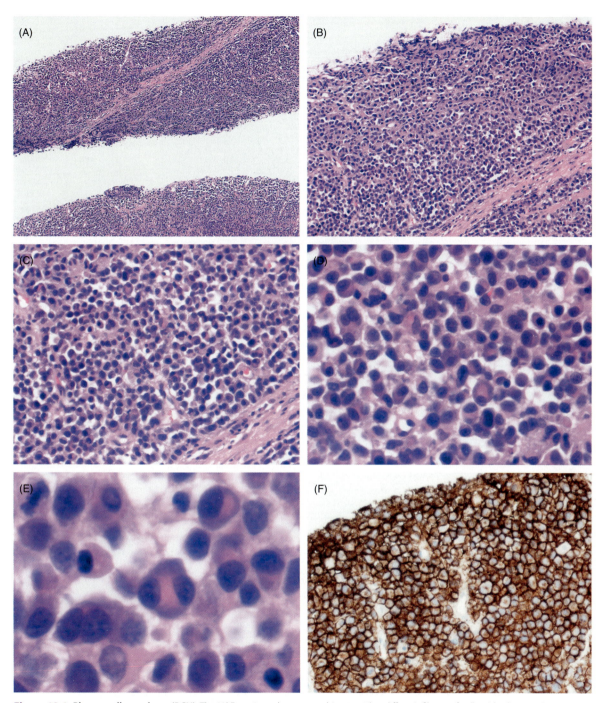

Figure 13.1 Plasma cell neoplasm (PCN). The H&E sections show a core biopsy with a diffuse infiltrate of cells with plasmacytic morphology (A–E). The cells show eosinophilic cytoplasm with a pale "hof" and eccentrically placed nuclei (C–E). Binucleate plasma cells are present (E). Immunohistochemistry shows strong positivity with CD138 (F), whilst both CD20 (G) and CD3 (H) are negative. The tumor cells were positive with MUM1/IRF4 and negative with CD56 and cyclin D1. The plasma cells show cytoplasmic kappa positivity (I) and are negative for lambda light chains (J).

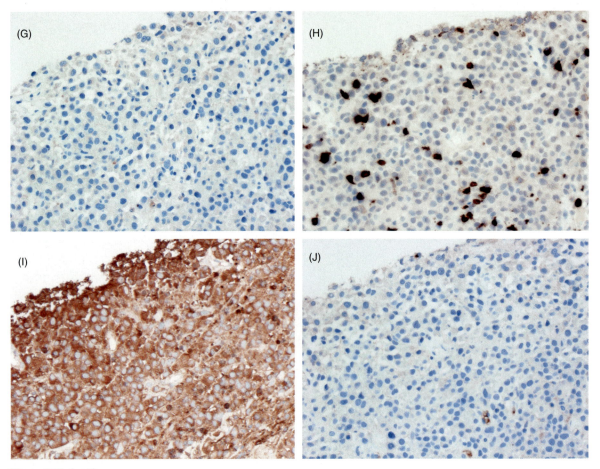

Figure 13.1 (cont.)

3. Plasmablastic lymphoma shows features that may overlap with diffuse large B cell lymphoma (DLBCL, see Chapter 9), particularly if the latter shows a degree of plasmacytic differentiation. PAX5 and CD20 expression favor DLBCL whereas expression of CD138, CD38 or VS38c support a diagnosis of plasmablastic lymphoma.

4. The tumor cells in primary effusion lymphoma (PEL) can show morphological features resembling plasmablasts.[21,22] Like plasmablastic lymphoma, PEL is often CD20 and CD79a negative and can express CD138, CD38 and VS38c. The diagnosis of PEL is confirmed by the detection of both HHV8 (LANA) and EBV (EBER) in the tumor cells.

5. Plasmablastic lymphoma can be confused with metastatic neoplasms such as melanoma or carcinoma (see below). Since plasmablastic lymphoma is often CD45 negative and can express cytokeratins there is the potential for a mistaken diagnosis of carcinoma. Where the lineage of a lesion is in question it is important to use an extended immunohistochemistry panel; light chain staining is critical in this situation.

Plasma cell neoplasms: problems and pitfalls of core biopsies

• Not all mature PCNs show the typical morphology. Some lesions are composed of small cells that resemble small lymphocytes. Where there is aberrant expression of CD20 the lesion may be misdiagnosed as a CD5 negative small B cell lymphoma. Lesions that are CD20 and

Table 13.1 Extended table of antibodies useful in the diagnosis of PCNs

Antibody	Specificity	Utility
CD138 (Syndecan)	Proteoglycan plasma cell marker	Positive staining in PCNs (also stains epithelial cells)
CD38	Cyclic ADP ribose hydrolase found on hemopoietic and lymphoid cells	Positive staining in PCNs
VS38c	Recognizes p63 on rough endoplasmic reticulum	Positive staining in mature plasma cells and in plasmacytic cells in PCNs and LPL
MUM1/IRF4	B cell proliferation and differentiation marker	Nuclear positivity in plasma cells
CD79a	B cell antigen receptor alpha chain	B lineage marker that stains a percentage of plasma cells
CD56	NCAM neural adhesion molecule	"Aberrant" marker positive in a subset of PCNs
Cyclin D1	Cyclin protein involved in cell cycle regulation, over-expressed in mantle cell lymphoma	Marks a subset of neoplastic plasma cells (some cases show a t(11;14) CCND1 translocation)
CD117	C-kit protein kinase expressed on common myeloid precursor cells	"Aberrant" marker positive in a subset of PCNs
CD20	Glycosylated phosphoprotein expressed on the surface of B cells	B lineage marker normally negative in plasma cells, but is positive in a subset of PCNs
PAX5	B cell marker – protein regulator expressed in early stages of B cell differentiation	B lineage marker that is negative in plasma cells
EBER	Epstein–Barr encoded viral RNAs	Positive in many plasmablastic lymphomas, particularly in the setting of HIV
IgG, IgM, IgA	Immunoglobulin heavy chains	Cytoplasmic staining in cells with plasmacytic differentiation
Kappa, lambda	Immunoglobulin light chains	Cytoplasmic staining in cells with plasmacytic differentiation

Abbreviations: HIV, human immunodeficiency virus; LPL, lymphoplasmacytic lymphoma; PCNs, plasma cell neoplasms.

cyclin D1 positive can be misdiagnosed as mantle cell lymphoma. Expression of CD138 and MUM1/IRF4 will correctly identify the cells as plasma cells.

- Beware of limited immunohistochemistry panels. Neoplastic plasma cells can show positivity with cytokeratins and EMA and can be CD45 negative. Conversely CD138 is positive on most carcinomas and can be expressed by malignant melanoma. The expression of T cell markers by PCNs can also lead to diagnostic confusion.[18] Light chains and PCR may be needed for the correct identification of a neoplastic plasma cell lesion.

- Although light chain staining is a key feature, neoplastic plasma cells may show very weak cytoplasmic positivity which can be difficult to distinguish from background non-specific staining. Good immunohistochemistry technique and close examination, with careful comparison of kappa and lambda, are required in this setting. As above, PCR may be needed in difficult cases.

References

1. Lorsbach RB, Hsi ED, Dogan A, Fend F. Plasma cell myeloma and related neoplasms. *Am J Clin Pathol* 2011;**136**:168–182.

2. Kilciksiz S, Karakoyun-Celik O, Agaoglu FY, Haydaroglu A. A review for solitary plasmacytoma of bone and extramedullary plasmacytoma. *Scientific World Journal* 2012;**2012**:895765.

3. Oriol A. Multiple myeloma with extramedullary disease. *Adv Ther* 2011;**28** Suppl 7:1–6.

4. Teruya-Feldstein J. Diffuse large B-cell lymphomas with plasmablastic differentiation. *Curr Oncol Rep* 2005;**7**:357–363.

5. Rafaniello Raviele P, Pruneri G, Maiorano E. Plasmablastic lymphoma: a review. *Oral Dis* 2009;**15**:38–45.

6. Castillo J, Pantanowitz L, Dezube BJ. HIV-associated plasmablastic lymphoma: lessons learned from 112 published cases. *Am J Hematol* 2008;**83**:804–809.

7. Carbone A, Cesarman E, Spina M, Gloghini A, Schulz TF. HIV-associated lymphomas and gamma-herpesviruses. *Blood* 2009;**113**:1213–1224.

8. Ruiz-Argüelles GJ, San Miguel JF. Cell surface markers in multiple myeloma. *Mayo Clin Proc* 1994;**69**:684–690.

9. Chilosi M, Adami F, Lestani M, et al. CD138/syndecan-1: a useful immunohistochemical marker of normal and neoplastic plasma cells on routine trephine bone marrow biopsies. *Mod Pathol* 1999;**12**:1101–1106.

10. Natkunam Y, Warnke RA, Montgomery K, Falini B, van De Rijn M. Analysis of MUM1/IRF4 protein expression using tissue microarrays and immunohistochemistry. *Mod Pathol* 2001;**14**:686–694.

11. Lin P, Mahdavy M, Zhan F, et al. Expression of PAX5 in CD20-positive multiple myeloma assessed by immunohistochemistry and oligonucleotide microarray. *Mod Pathol* 2004;**17**:1217–1222.

12. Haghighi B, Yanagihara R, Cornbleet PJ. IgM myeloma: case report with immunophenotypic profile. *Am J Hematol* 1998;**59**:302–308.

13. Van Camp B, Durie BG, Spier C, et al. Plasma cells in multiple myeloma express a natural killer cell-associated antigen: CD56 (NKH-1; Leu-19). *Blood* 1990;**76**:377–382.

14. Maiso P, Ghobrial IM. Would the real myeloma cell please stand up? *Leuk Lymphoma* 2012;**53**:1851–1852.

15. Pozdnyakova O, Morgan EA, Li B, Shahsafaei A, Dorfman DM. Patterns of expression of CD56 and CD117 on neoplastic plasma cells and association with genetically distinct subtypes of plasma cell myeloma. *Leuk Lymphoma* 2012;**53**:1905–1910.

16. Vasef MA, Medeiros LJ, Yospur LS, et al. Cyclin D1 protein in multiple myeloma and plasmacytoma: an immunohistochemical study using fixed, paraffin-embedded tissue sections. *Mod Pathol* 1997;**10**:927–932.

17. Yeung J, Chang H. Genomic aberrations and immunohistochemical markers as prognostic indicators in multiple myeloma. *J Clin Pathol* 2008;**61**:832–836.

18. Spier CM, Grogan TM, Durie BG, et al. T-cell antigen-positive multiple myeloma. *Mod Pathol* 1990;**3**:302–307.

19. Wotherspoon AC, Norton AJ, Isaacson PG. Immunoreactive cytokeratins in plasmacytomas. *Histopathology* 1989;**14**:141–150.

20. Pangalis GA, Angelopoulou MK, Vassilakopoulos TP, Siakantaris MP, Kittas C. B-chronic lymphocytic leukemia, small lymphocytic lymphoma, and lymphoplasmacytic lymphoma, including Waldenström's macroglobulinemia: a clinical, morphologic, and biologic spectrum of similar disorders. *Semin Hematol* 1999;**36**:104–114.

21. Gaidano G, Carbone A. Primary effusion lymphoma: a liquid phase lymphoma of fluid-filled body cavities. *Adv Cancer Res* 2001;**80**:115–146.

22. Montes-Moreno S, Montalbán C, Piris MA. Large B-cell lymphomas with plasmablastic differentiation: a biological and therapeutic challenge. *Leuk Lymphoma* 2012;**53**:185–194.

Illustrative cases: Plasma cell neoplasms

13

Illustrative case 1

History: Female aged 85 who presented with shortness of breath, fatigue and generalized lymphadenopathy. Computed tomography (CT) showed significantly enlarged lymph nodes in the cervical region, mediastinum, axilla, pelvis and groin. Core biopsy of left femoral lymph node.

Comments: The biopsy shows effacement of the normal nodal architecture by a pleomorphic cellular infiltrate. Many of the cells show abundant pale cytoplasm with an eccentrically placed nucleus giving the tumor a "signet ring" appearance. The tumor cells are CD45 and CD79a positive. CD138 is expressed by most of the cells with

signet ring morphology and CD20 stains only scattered cells. CD3 is negative and there is nuclear expression of MUM1/IRF4. There is cytoplasmic IgG positivity and kappa light chain restriction. EBER staining is negative and MIB1 shows a proliferation fraction of 60–70%.

The infiltrate here shows prominent nuclear atypia accompanying a signet ring morphology, so the differential diagnosis includes metastatic signet ring carcinoma. CD45 confirms a lymphoid lineage and CD79a confirms a B cell neoplasm. Plasmacytic differentiation is indicated by CD138 and MUM1/IRF4 positivity and cytoplasmic expression of IgG and kappa light chains. CD20 is negative in the majority of the tumor cells, but scattered cells have retained positivity.

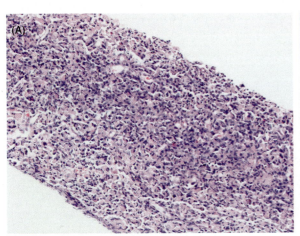 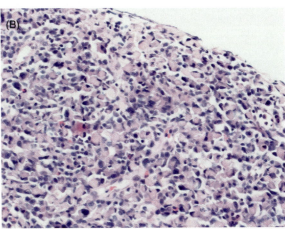

Illustrative case 1 (A–D) H&E sections show a diffuse infiltrate of atypical cells, many of which have abundant pale cytoplasm with the nucleus displaced to the periphery of the cell to give a signet ring appearance. At high power (C,D) many of the cells have hyperchromatic pleomorphic nuclei and some admixed eosinophils are noted. The tumor cells are CD45 positive (E), confirming a lymphoma and excluding signet ring carcinoma. CD79a is strongly positive (F) and the cells with signet ring morphology are seen to express CD138 (G). CD20 is largely negative (H), although occasional signet ring cells are positive. CD3 stains background T lymphocytes (I) and the tumor cells show strong nuclear expression of MUM1/IRF4 (J). The pale cytoplasm of the signet ring cells contains immunoglobulin; there is cytoplasmic expression of IgG (K) and kappa light chains (L).

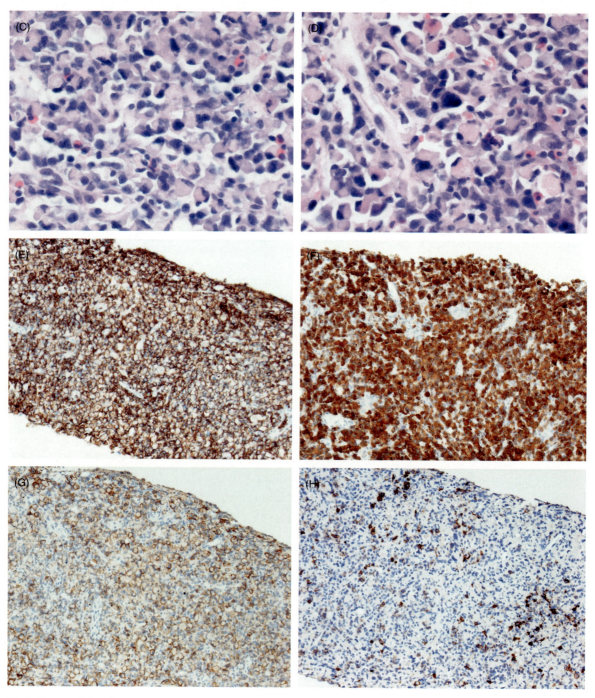

Illustrative case 1 (cont.)

The features here, including the nuclear pleomorphism and high proliferation fraction with MIB1, are those of a high grade B cell lymphoma with prominent plasma cell differentiation which could be categorized either as an anaplastic plasma cell neoplasm or a plasmablastic lymphoma. A bone marrow trephine biopsy showed no evidence of plasma cell myeloma, and the patient was treated for a systemic plasmablastic lymphoma.

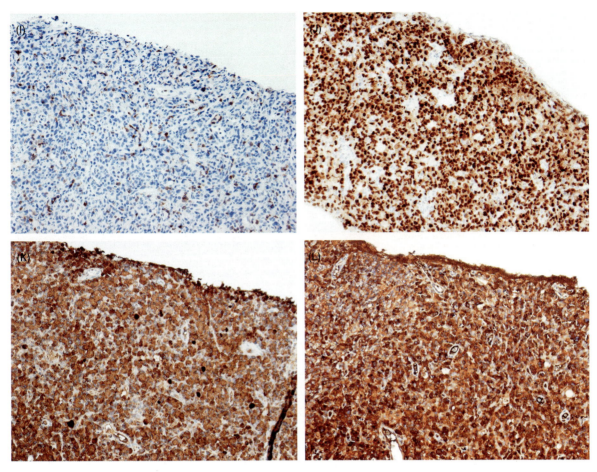

Illustrative case 1 (cont.)

Illustrative case 2

History: Female aged 76 with generalized lymphadenopathy. Core biopsy from lymph node in left groin region.

Comments: The normal nodal structure is replaced by extensive deposits of amorphous eosinophilic material within which are prominent dilated blood vessels. The amorphous material is Congo Red positive and shows areas of green dichroic birefringence under polarized light. Scattered groups of small lymphocytes and plasma cells are present.

The lymphocytes are a mixture of T and B cells. The plasma cells are CD138 positive and show kappa light chain restriction.

The picture is that of primary amyloidosis. There is extensive deposition of amyloid material that shows the typical Congo Red positivity and "apple-green" birefringence. Although relatively few plasma cells are present, there is distinct kappa light chain restriction and a suggestion of kappa positivity within the amyloid material itself. The plasma cells were CD56 and cyclin D1 negative. Nodal involvement is rare in primary amyloidosis.

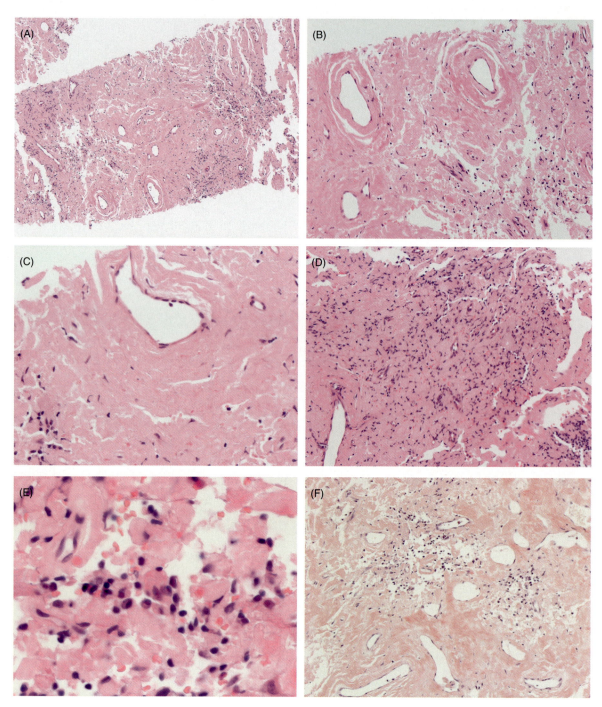

Illustrative case 2 (A–C) Routine H&E stains show that the normal lymph node architecture is completely obliterated by sheets of pale eosinophilic material. The material is amorphous and surrounds prominent dilated blood vessels (B,C). Scattered groups of lymphocytes and plasma cells are present within the eosinophilic material (D,E). The amorphous material is positive with Congo Red staining (F) and under polarized light shows focal areas which have a bright green birefringence (G). CD138 stains the plasma cells (H); the lymphocytes were a mixture of T and B cells (not shown). The plasma cells show prominent cytoplasmic positivity with kappa light chains (I) and are negative for lambda light chains (J).

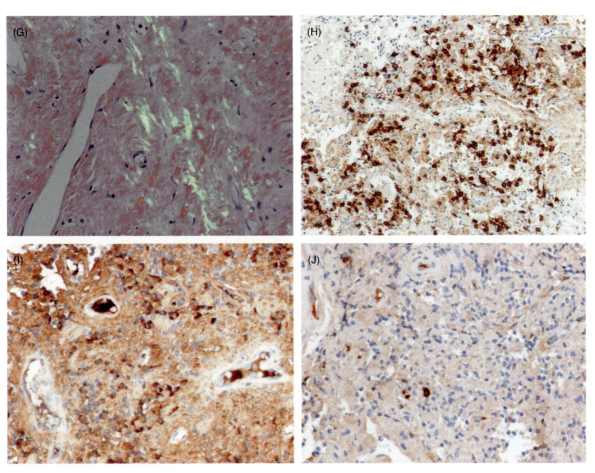

Illustrative case 2 (cont.)

Other pathology seen in lymph node needle core biopsies

Although the majority of needle core biopsies will demonstrate pathology that would fall into the overall category of "lymphoid," specimens can contain a variety of other conditions. These may fall outside the area of expertise of the hematopathologist, and where the lesion can be classified it is advisable to consult with an appropriate specialist. This section presents a brief overview of some of these conditions and provides outline guidance of how they can be handled, at least in the first instance. Table 14.1 provides a broad, but not comprehensive, list of antibodies that may be required to investigate biopsies in this category.

One particular category of lesion that can cause problems is that of hematopathological disease falling outside the usual spectrum of reactive and neoplastic lymphoid proliferations. This group includes myeloid sarcoma and rare histiocytic and dendritic cell lesions. Myeloid sarcoma can be a particular diagnostic problem.[1,2] The lesions of myeloid sarcoma may morphologically resemble a lymphoma (Fig. 14.1A–C) and express CD45 (Fig. 14.1D). There may be no clinical history of myeloid leukemia or myelodysplasia. Lymphoid lineage markers such as CD20 and CD3 will be negative (Fig. 14.1E, F). In this setting a wide range of myeloid and monocytic antibodies (Table 14.1) are available. CD68 will usually show positivity in at least some of the tumor cells (Fig. 14.1G), lysozyme is frequently positive (Fig. 14.1H) and there will be variable expression of other myelomonocytic antigens. There is often monocytic differentiation, so CD34 is generally negative. Helpful myeloid markers include CD33, MPO, CD15, and CD13. More monocytic/monoblastic lesions may stain with CD11c (Fig. 14.1I), CD163, HLA-DR and CD4.[1–4] Some examples will express CD123 indicating plasmacytoid dendritic cell differentiation.[5] There can be a phenotypic overlap with true histiocytic neoplasms. Rare cases of histiocytic sarcoma will express similar monocytic antigens but tend to show greater nuclear pleomorphism.[6,7] Langerhans cell histiocytosis shows the characteristic cellular morphology, with irregular "twisted" and grooved nuclei, prominent

pale eosinophilic cytoplasm and frequent associated eosinophils. The neoplastic Langerhans cells express S100, CD1a and Langerin (CD207) as well as CD68, HLA-DR and CD4.[8,9] Rare examples of interdigitating dendritic cell sarcoma will also express S100, but are Langerin and CD1a negative.[9,10] Follicular dendritic cell sarcomas can morphologically resemble soft tissue tumors and will variably express the follicular dendritic cell markers CD21, CD23 and CD35 as well as desmoplakin and fascin.[10,11]

Metastatic disease makes up the other broad group in this category. Core biopsies may contain metastases from a variety of tumor types arising at almost any site in the body. The overall approach is to classify the lesion as carcinoma, melanoma, germ cell tumor or sarcoma and, where possible, to identify a subcategory that will indicate a likely primary site. The basic features of each of these tumor categories are listed below.

- Metastatic carcinoma can show a wide variety of histological appearances. The cells are generally cohesive and often show an associated stromal fibrous reaction (Fig. 14.2A) or necrosis. Tumor cells may show clear or eosinophilic (Fig. 14.2B,C) cytoplasm. Nuclei are pleomorphic, nucleoli are often prominent and mitotic figures are often common. Keratinization may be seen in metastatic squamous cell carcinoma (Fig. 14.2D). Pancytokeratin staining is positive (Fig. 14.2E), and specific cytokeratins including CK5 (Fig. 14.2F), CK7 and CK20 can help in determining the likely primary site (Table 14.1). P63 (Fig. 14.2G) or p40 staining are markers of a squamous origin and TTF1 marks lung adenocarcinoma. Some small cell lung carcinomas will be negative for cytokeratins but are normally positive for CD56 and TTF1.[12,13]
- The morphology of metastatic melanoma is highly protean, with cohesive clusters of cells showing rounded, oval or spindle-shaped outlines (Fig. 14.3A–E). Cytoplasm is usually prominent

Table 14.1 Summary table of antibodies useful in the diagnosis of non-lymphomatous neoplasms in needle core biopsies

Antibody	Specificity	Utility
CD45	Leukocyte common antigen – membrane glycoprotein expressed on all hemopoietic and lymphoid cells	Positive staining indicates a hematolymphoid origin. Negative in some lymphomas, but false positives are very rare
CD117	C-kit protein kinase expressed on common myeloid precursor cells	Positive in primitive myelomonocytic cells; may be seen in myeloid sarcoma. Also expressed in mast cells, some epithelial malignancies and gastro-intestinal stromal tumors
CD68 (KP1 and PGM1)	Glycoprotein that binds to low density lipoprotein and is expressed on monocytes and macrophages	Granular cytoplasmic positivity in most cases of myeloid sarcoma
MPO	Peroxidase enzyme expressed abundantly in granulocytic cells	Positive in some myeloid sarcoma cases
CD13	Aminopeptidase expressed in granulocytes, monocytes and a number of epithelial cells	Positive in some myeloid sarcoma cases
CD15	Carbohydrate adhesion molecule expressed in mature granulocytes	Positive in some myeloid sarcoma cases; expressed in Reed–Sternberg cells in classical Hodgkin lymphoma
CD33	Transmembrane receptor expressed on cells of myeloid and monocytic lineage	Positive in some myeloid sarcoma cases
CD11c	Integrin protein expressed on monocytes and macrophages	Stains normal histiocytes and cases of myeloid sarcoma with monocytic differentiation
CD163	Hemoglobin scavenger receptor found on cells of monocyte/macrophage lineage	Stains normal histiocytes and cases of myeloid sarcoma with monocytic differentiation
Lysozyme	Muramidase glycoside hydrolase present in the granules of neutrophils	Granular cytoplasmic positivity in some cases of myeloid sarcoma
AE1/AE3	Cocktail of anti-cytokeratin antibodies	"Pan" cytokeratin – broad spectrum marker of epithelial malignancies
CK5	High molecular weight cytokeratin	Predictive of a primary tumor of squamous epithelial origin
CK7 and CK20	Cytokeratins differentially expressed on metastatic carcinomas of glandular origin	• Gastric, biliary, mucinous ovarian, pancreatic and urothelial carcinomas are CK7 positive and CK20 positive • Breast, endometrial, serous ovarian and lung carcinomas are CK7 positive and CK20 negative • Colorectal, gastric and Merkel cell carcinomas are CK7 negative and CK20 positive • Hepatocellular, prostatic, renal cell, thyroid, small cell lung, squamous esophageal and squamous lung carcinomas are CK7 negative and CK20 negative
CK19	Acidic cytokeratin	Positive in thymic epithelium, papillary carcinoma of thyroid and carcinomas of pancreas, gastro-intestinal tract and liver
p63	Transcription factor in the p53 family	Nuclear positivity supports a primary tumor of squamous epithelial origin
p40	Recognizes an isoform of p63 reported to be more specific for squamous or basal cells	Nuclear positivity supports a primary tumor of squamous epithelial origin
TTF1	Thyroid transcription factor 1; gene regulator protein in thyroid and lung cells	Marks thyroid carcinoma and small cell carcinoma and adenocarcinoma of the lung
CD56	NCAM neural adhesion molecule	Expressed in neuroendocrine carcinomas and small cell lung carcinoma, as well as a number of lymphoid malignancies
S100	Protein expressed in cells derived from the neural crest, macrophages, dendritic cells and Langerhans cells	Positive in metastatic melanoma some neural sarcomas
HMB45	Antigen extracted from melanoma cells	Marks metastatic malignant melanoma
Melan-A	Protein antigen present on the surface of melanocytes	Marks metastatic malignant melanoma

Table 14.1 (cont.)

Antibody	Specificity	Utility
PLAP	Placental alkaline phosphatase	Marks metastatic seminoma
OCT-3/4	Transcription factor important in pluripotent germ cells	Nuclear positivity in seminoma and embryonal carcinoma
D2–40	Podoplanin; transmembrane mucoprotein expressed by lymphatic epithelium and seminoma cells	Marks metastatic seminoma
CD30	Cell membrane protein of the tumor necrosis factor receptor family	Marker of embryonal carcinoma as well as Hodgkin/Reed–Sternberg (HRS) cells, activated lymphoid cells and some melanomas
Desmin	Intermediate filament subunit found in skeletal, smooth and cardiac muscle tissue	Marker of muscle differentiation – positive in myogenic and myofibroblastic tumors
SMA (ASMA)	Alpha smooth muscle actin	Marker of myofibroblasts and smooth muscle cells
HHV8 (LANA)	Latency-associated nuclear antigen of HHV8	Nuclear positivity in Kaposi sarcoma and in HHV8-related lymphomas

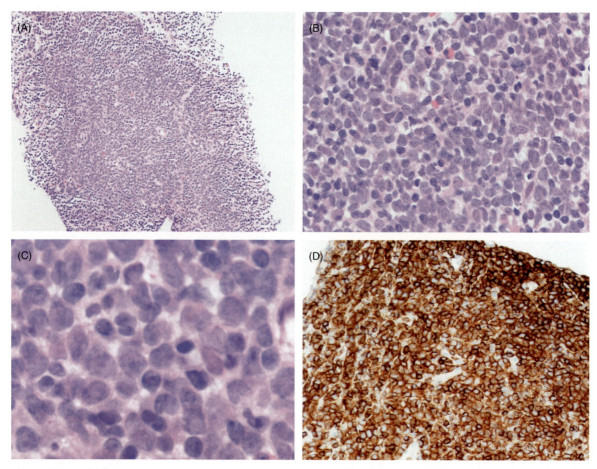

Figure 14.1 Myeloid sarcoma. Core biopsy showing an infiltrate of monomorphic cells with pale slightly irregular nuclei, single or multiple eosinophilic nuclei and little cytoplasm (A–C, H&E). The morphological appearance suggests a lymphoma, and the tumor cells are CD45 positive (D). CD20 is negative (E) and CD3 shows a background T cell population (F). A sub-population of the tumor cell show granular cytoplasmic positivity for CD68 (G) and lysozyme (H), and there is widespread expression of CD11c (I).

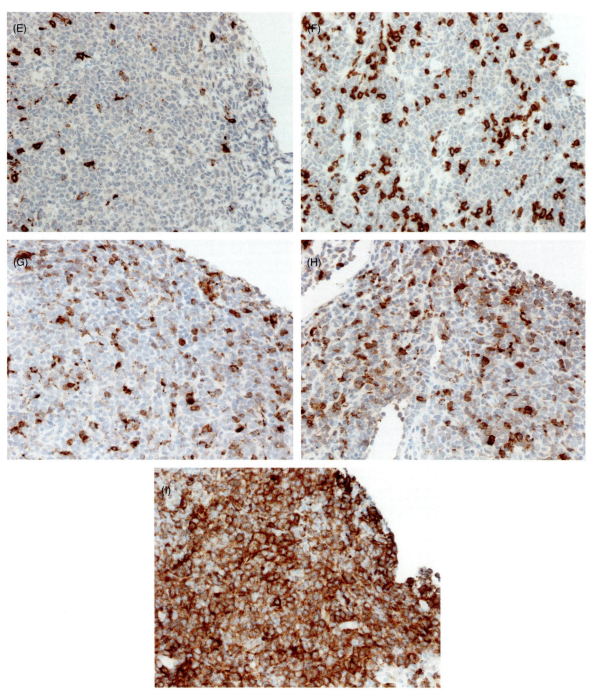

Figure 14.1 (cont.)

and eosinophilic and the nuclei may show large eosinophilic nuclei or pale inclusions (Fig. 14.3D). Mitotic activity is high and melanin pigment can be seen in some cases (Fig. 14.3C–E), although a number of cases are amelanotic. Immunohistochemistry will confirm the diagnosis; melanoma cells are positive with S100 (Fig. 14.3F), HMB45 (Fig. 14.3G) and melan-A (Fig. 14.3H).[14]

147

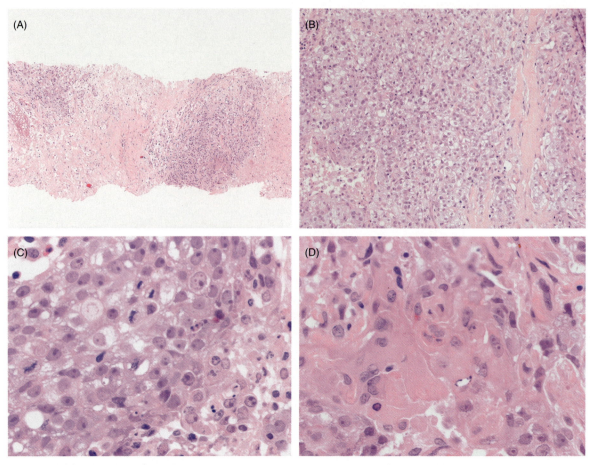

Figure 14.2 Metastatic squamous cell carcinoma. Low power H&E shows replacement of the normal lymphoid tissue by sclerotic nodules of tumor (A). The tumor contains cohesive sheets of clear cells and cells with eosinophilic cytoplasm (B). High power shows pleomorphic rounded nuclei, prominent eosinophilic nucleoli, eosinophilic and clear cytoplasm and frequent mitoses (C). Focal areas of keratinization are present (D). The tumor cells express AE1/AE3 (E), CK5 (F) and p63 (G).

- Metastatic germ cell tumors, in particular seminoma, may mimic lymphoma. The infiltrating cells are often monomorphic and have rounded nuclei that resemble centroblasts or immunoblasts (Fig. 14.4A–D). These cells show greater cohesion than in diffuse large B cell lymphoma, frequently forming small clusters, and the cytoplasm is clear and vacuolated (Fig. 14.4C,D). CD45 will be negative, although there is often a background lymphoid population (Fig. 14.4E). Cytokeratins and melanoma markers such as S100 (Fig. 14.4F) will be negative. PLAP and OCT-3/4 are positive (Fig. 14.4G,H).[15,16]

- Metastatic sarcoma is rare in needle core biopsies. Tumor cells may be spindle-shaped (Fig. 14.5A–D) or epithelioid. CD45 will usually be negative and many, but not all, cases will be cytokeratin negative (for example, biphasic synovial sarcomas will show focal cytokeratin positivity). S100 may be positive in neural sarcomas, but HMB45 and melan-A will be negative. Desmin and SMA staining may indicate muscle differentiation and endothelial markers (CD31, CD34) can reveal an endothelial origin. Occasional specific tumor types will show characteristic markers, such as HHV8 staining in Kaposi sarcoma (Fig. 14.5E).[17]

One final category of specimen that is often difficult to diagnose is core biopsies coming from patients whose lymphomas have been treated. The clinical teams are usually looking for either residual (unresponsive) disease or a recurrence of the original

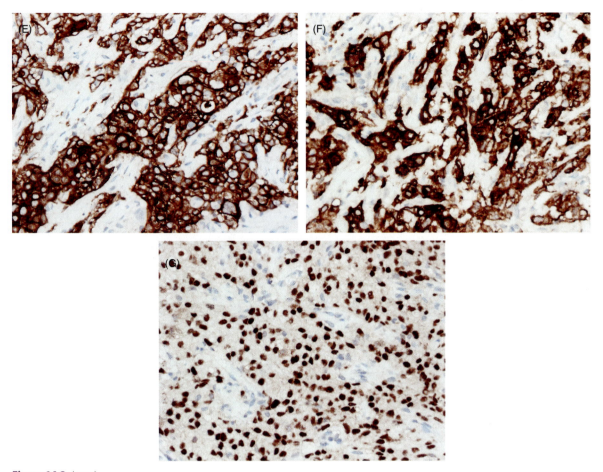

Figure 14.2 (cont.)

tumor. Such specimens will show the histological effects of chemotherapy, which can include partial or complete necrosis, fibrin deposition, fibrosis and a histiocytic reaction. Immunohistochemistry is often required to exclude lymphoma; necrotic cells may retain antigens such as CD20, CD3, CD30 and CD138.[18,19] Patients being treated for lymphoma or leukemia may be neutropenic, and staining for fungal infections or acid-fast bacteria are recommended, particularly if the biopsy contains sheets of histiocytes.

Differential diagnosis

1. Anaplastic large cell lymphoma (ALCL). The pleomorphic nature of the cells in ALCL may resemble those of a poorly differentiated carcinoma or melanoma.[20,21] ALCL cells frequently show a partly cohesive sinusoidal pattern reminiscent of metastatic carcinoma. In addition, some ALCL cases are CD45 negative and may lack expression of T lineage markers (the "null-cell" phenotype). CD30 positivity will indicate ALCL, but is not diagnostic (see below). Absence of staining with cytokeratins and melanoma markers is helpful, and strong expression of cytotoxic markers (perforin, granzyme B and TIA1) will help identify ALCL. Cytokeratin positivity has been recorded in ALCL.[22]

2. Plasmablastic lymphoma. Highly pleomorphic plasma cell tumors can be morphologically similar to metastatic melanoma or carcinoma. Since plasmablastic lymphomas are often CD45 negative, and since metastatic carcinoma (and melanoma) can express CD138, there is a potential

149

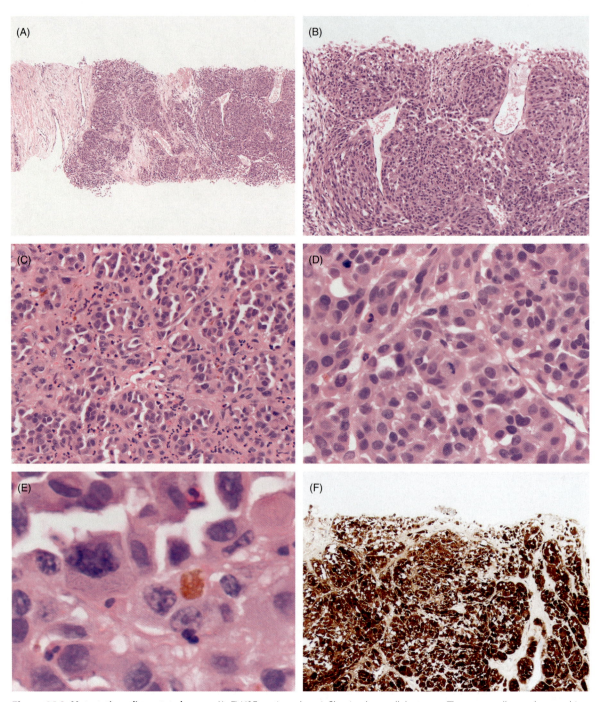

Figure 14.3 Metastatic malignant melanoma. (A–E) H&E sections show infiltration by a cellular tumor. The tumor cells are pleomorphic and have eosinophilic cytoplasm, frequent mitoses and pale nuclear inclusions (C,D). Melanin pigment is present in scattered tumor cells (C,E). There is positive staining with S100 (F), HMB45 (G) and melan-A (H).

for diagnostic confusion.[23] Occasional plasma cell neoplasms can show aberrant cytokeratin expression. MUM1/IRF4 is often helpful, and identifying immunoglobulin light chain production will confirm a diagnosis of plasmablastic lymphoma. Polymerase chain

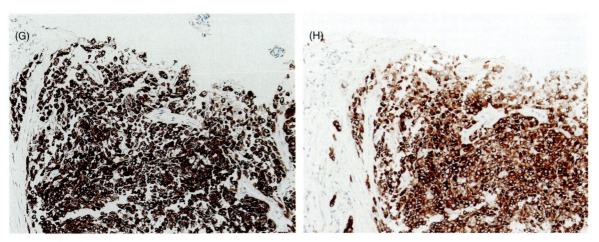

Figure 14.3 (cont.)

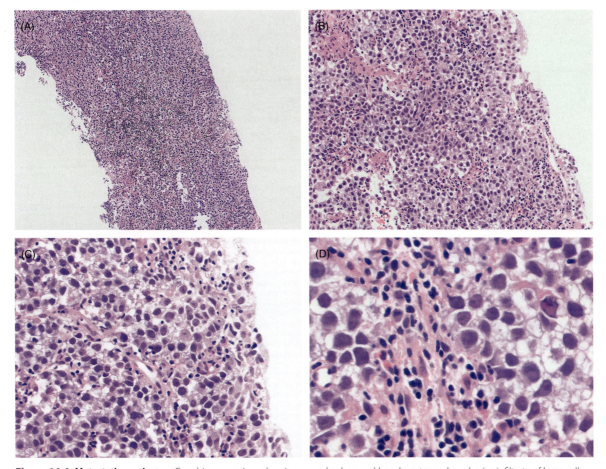

Figure 14.4 Metastatic seminoma. Core biopsy sections showing some background lymphocytes and a cohesive infiltrate of large cells with rounded nuclei, prominent nucleoli and clear partly vacuolated cytoplasm (A–D, H&E). The high power view (D) shows scattered small lymphocytes amongst the tumor cells. The tumor cells are negative with CD45 (E) and HMB45 (F) but are strongly positive with PLAP (G) and OCT-3/4 (H).

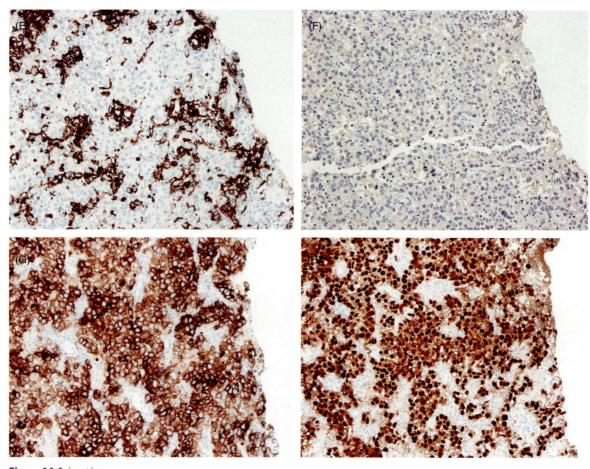

Figure 14.4 (cont.)

reaction (PCR) for B cell clonality may be required in difficult cases.

3. Biopsies from thymoma may be mistaken for T lymphoblastic leukemia/lymphoma. Cytokeratins are required to identify the epithelial component of a thymoma.[24]

Other neoplasms: problems and pitfalls of core biopsies

- Whilst CD45 is a reliable marker of lymphoid and hematological cells and false positives are extremely rare, some lymphomas are negative with this marker. ALCL, plasmablastic lymphoma, primary effusion lymphoma, and classical Hodgkin lymphoma are all frequently CD45 negative.

- CD138 marks plasma cells, but is also positive on many epithelial tumors and on malignant melanoma.[23]

- CD30 is positive in ALCL, but metastatic embryonal carcinoma and metastatic malignant melanoma can also express this marker. Metastatic seminoma can also express CD10.[25]

- Metastatic non-lymphoid neoplasms will often contain a large number of intra-tumoral histiocytes. Staining such tumors with macrophage markers may incorrectly suggest a histiocytic origin, especially in small biopsies containing a limited amount of tumor. Close examination of these macrophage markers (and sometimes CD45) is required in order to determine if the neoplastic cells are truly positive.

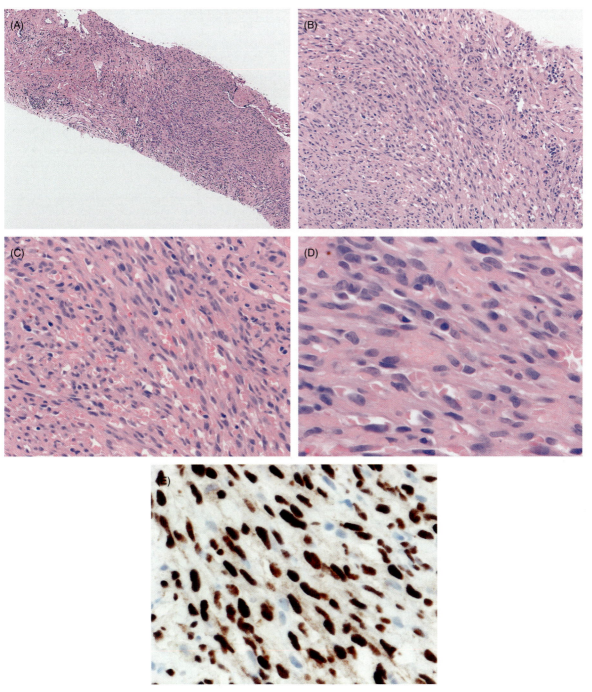

Figure 14.5 Kaposi sarcoma. The sections show a core biopsy from a human immunodeficiency virus (HIV)-positive patient with nodal Kaposi sarcoma. At low power (A) the lymphoid tissue has been replaced by an infiltrate of spindle-shaped cells. Higher power H&E sections (B–D) show eosinophilic spindle cells with intervening irregular vascular spaces. Scattered plasma cells are also present (C,D). The tumor cell nuclei stain positively for HHV8 (LANA) (E).

References

1. Audouin J, Comperat E, Le Tourneau A, et al. Myeloid sarcoma: clinical and morphologic criteria useful for diagnosis. *Int J Surg Pathol* 2003;**11**:271–282.

2. Campidelli C, Agostinelli C, Stitson R, Pileri SA. Myeloid sarcoma: extramedullary manifestation of myeloid disorders. *Am J Clin Pathol* 2009;**132**:426–437.

3. Klco JM, Welch JS, Nguyen TT, et al. State of the art in myeloid sarcoma. *Int J Lab Hematol* 2011;**33**:555–565.

4. Hoyer JD, Grogg KL, Hanson CA, Gamez JD, Dogan A. CD33 detection by immunohistochemistry in paraffin-embedded tissues: a new antibody shows excellent specificity and sensitivity for cells of myelomonocytic lineage. *Am J Clin Pathol* 2008;**129**:316–323.

5. Alexiev BA, Wang W, Ning Y, et al. Myeloid sarcomas: a histologic, immunohistochemical, and cytogenetic study. *Diagn Pathol* 2007;**2**:42.

6. Copie-Bergman C, Wotherspoon AC, Norton AJ, Diss TC, Isaacson PG. True histiocytic lymphoma: a morphologic, immunohistochemical, and molecular genetic study of 13 cases. *Am J Surg Pathol* 1998;**22**:1386–1392.

7. Yoshida C, Takeuchi M. Histiocytic sarcoma: identification of its histiocytic origin using immunohistochemistry. *Intern Med* 2008;**47**:165–169.

8. Edelweiss M, Medeiros LJ, Suster S, Moran CA. Lymph node involvement by Langerhans cell histiocytosis: a clinicopathologic and immunohistochemical study of 20 cases. *Hum Pathol* 2007;**38**:1463–1469.

9. Lau SK, Chu PG, Weiss LM. Immunohistochemical expression of Langerin in Langerhans cell histiocytosis and non-Langerhans cell histiocytic disorders. *Am J Surg Pathol* 2008;**32**:615–619.

10. Pileri SA, Grogan TM, Harris NL, et al. Tumours of histiocytes and accessory dendritic cells: an immunohistochemical approach to classification from the International Lymphoma Study Group based on 61 cases. *Histopathology* 2002;**41**:1–29.

11. Kairouz S, Hashash J, Kabbara W, McHayleh W, Tabbara IA. Dendritic cell neoplasms: an overview. *Am J Hematol* 2007;**82**:924–928.

12. Mukhopadhyay S, Katzenstein AL. Subclassification of non-small cell lung carcinomas lacking morphologic differentiation on biopsy specimens: utility of an immunohistochemical panel containing TTF-1, napsin A, p63, and CK5/6. *Am J Surg Pathol* 2011;**35**:15–25.

13. Nobre AR, Albergaria A, Schmitt F. p40: a p63 isoform useful for lung cancer diagnosis – a review of the physiological and pathological role of p63. *Acta Cytol* 2013;**57**:1–8.

14. Ferringer T. Update on immunohistochemistry in melanocytic lesions. *Dermatol Clin* 2012;**30**:567–579.

15. Leroy X, Augusto D, Leteurtre E, Gosselin B. CD30 and CD117 (c-kit) used in combination are useful for distinguishing embryonal carcinoma from seminoma. *J Histochem Cytochem* 2002;**50**:283–285.

16. Iczkowski KA, Butler SL, Shanks JH, et al. Trials of new germ cell immunohistochemical stains in 93 extragonadal and metastatic germ cell tumors. *Hum Pathol* 2008;**39**:275–281.

17. Komatsu T, Barbera AJ, Ballestas ME, Kaye KM. The Kaposi's sarcoma-associated herpesvirus latency-associated nuclear antigen. *Viral Immunol* 2001;**14**:311–317.

18. Norton AJ, Ramsay AD, Isaacson PG. Antigen preservation in infarcted lymphoid tissue. A novel approach to the infarcted lymph node using monoclonal antibodies effective in routinely processed tissues. *Am J Surg Pathol* 1988;**12**:759–767.

19. Kojima M, Nakamura S, Yamane Y, et al. Antigen preservation in infarcted nodal B-cell lymphoma, with special reference to follicular center cell markers. *Int J Surg Pathol* 2004;**12**:251–255.

20. Foss RD, Laskin WB, Lombardi DP, Morton AL, Snyder J. Anaplastic large cell lymphoma. *Head Neck* 1991;**13**:545–548.

21. Pulitzer M, Brady MS, Blochin E, Amin B, Teruya-Feldstein J. Anaplastic large cell lymphoma: a potential pitfall in the differential diagnosis of melanoma. *Arch Pathol Lab Med* 2013;**137**:280–283.

22. Zhang Q, Ming J, Zhang S, et al. Cytokeratin positivity in anaplastic large cell lymphoma: a potential diagnostic pitfall in misdiagnosis of metastatic carcinoma. *Int J Clin Exp Pathol* 2013;**6**:798–801.

23. O'Connell FP, Pinkus JL, Pinkus GS. CD138 (syndecan-1), a plasma cell marker immunohistochemical profile in hematopoietic and nonhematopoietic neoplasms. *Am J Clin Pathol* 2004;**121**:254–263.

24. Hasserjian RP, Ströbel P, Marx A. Pathology of thymic tumors. *Semin Thorac Cardiovasc Surg* 2005;**17**:2–11.

25. Ota Y, Iihara K, Ryu T, Morikawa T, Fukayama M. Metastatic seminomas in lymph nodes: CD10 immunoreactivity can be a pitfall of differential diagnosis. *Int J Clin Exp Pathol* 2013;**6**:498–502.

26. Chilosi M, Castelli P, Martignoni G, et al. Neoplastic epithelial cells in a subset of human thymomas express the B cell-associated CD20 antigen. *Am J Surg Pathol* 1992;**16**:988–997.

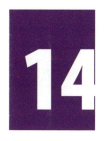

14 Illustrative cases: Other pathology seen in lymph node needle core biopsies

Illustrative case 1

History: Male aged 54. History of plasma cell myeloma treated with an autologous stem cell transplant. Patient diagnosed with relapsed disease and now on chemotherapy. The patient developed enlarged cervical nodes suspicious for transformation to a high grade tumor. Core biopsy from one of these nodes.

Comments: The picture is that of a plasma cell neoplasm showing the effects of chemotherapy. Although the

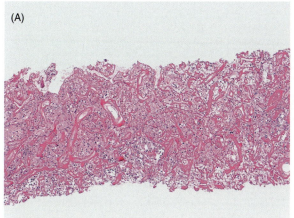

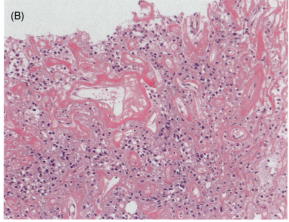

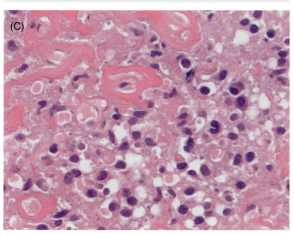

Illustrative case 1 (A–C) H&E sections show partly necrotic tissue with prominent fibrin deposition around blood vessels. Scattered viable cells are present, some with plasmacytic morphology (C). CD138 shows widespread positivity confirming a plasma cell infiltrate (D). The plasma cells are CD56 positive (E). There is cytoplasmic kappa positivity (F) and lambda light chain staining is negative (G).

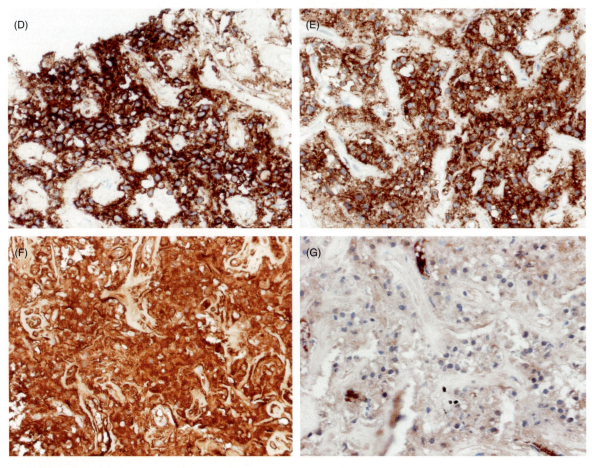

Illustrative case 1 (cont.)

morphology is not fully diagnostic, CD138 stains both viable and necrotic plasma cells. The plasma cells are CD56 positive and there is kappa light chain restriction.

Although tumor necrosis following chemotherapy can make interpretation difficult, the necrotic cells often retain many of their normal antigens, so immunohistochemistry will enable a positive diagnosis.

Illustrative case 2

History: Male aged 73. The patient had suffered from chronic lymphocytic leukemia/small lymphocytic lymphoma for 20 years and has had treatment with multiple chemotherapy regimens and immunosuppressive antibodies. He presented with swelling of left side of the face over several months. Scans showed a partly necrotic enhancing lesion in the left infratemporal fossa. Clinically this was thought to be necrotic transformed chronic lymphocytic leukemia. A first biopsy showed only fibrovascular tissue and skeletal muscle, so this repeat biopsy was performed.

Comments: The histology here shows fibromuscular tissue and several foci of necrosis with some scattered lymphoid cells. Within the necrosis there are numerous fungal hyphae. The fungal walls are positive with Grocott methenamine silver and periodic acid–Schiff stains. The hyphae are septate and branch in a dichotomous fashion. There is no evidence of chronic lymphocytic leukemia or transformation.

Post-chemotherapy complications include neutropenia and immunosuppression, with an increased risk of fungal infections. The morphology here is consistent with *Aspergillosis* infection, but histology is not fully diagnostic and other fungal species are possible.

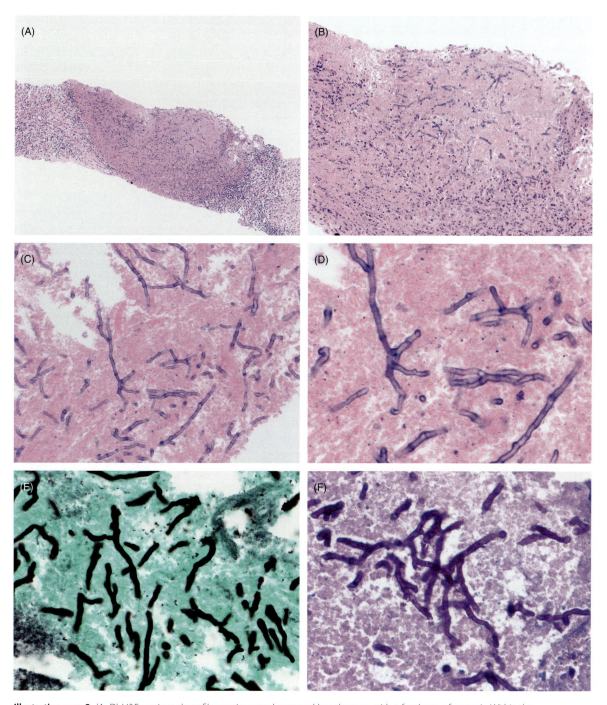

Illustrative case 2 (A–D) H&E sections show fibrous tissue and scattered lymphocytes with a focal area of necrosis. Within the necrotic region there is nuclear debris and multiple fungal hyphae. At high power the hyphae are septate and show dichotomous branching (C,D). The fungi are positive with Grocott (E) and PAS (F) stains.

Illustrative case 3

History: Female aged 64. Presented with a mediastinal "lymph node" mass which was biopsied. Thymoma was the most likely clinical diagnosis, but lymphoma and teratoma had to be excluded.

Comments: The clinical diagnosis here was correct, so the biopsy did not present a diagnostic problem.

Where the epithelial cells are subtle (and cytokeratin staining omitted), the presence of TdT-positive T cells with a high proliferation rate and the morphology of lymphoblasts can be mistaken for lymphoblastic leukemia/lymphoma (LBL – see Chapter 11). Cytokeratin staining shows the characteristic thymic epithelial network; the expression of CD20 by epithelial cells is a well-recognized feature of thymomas.

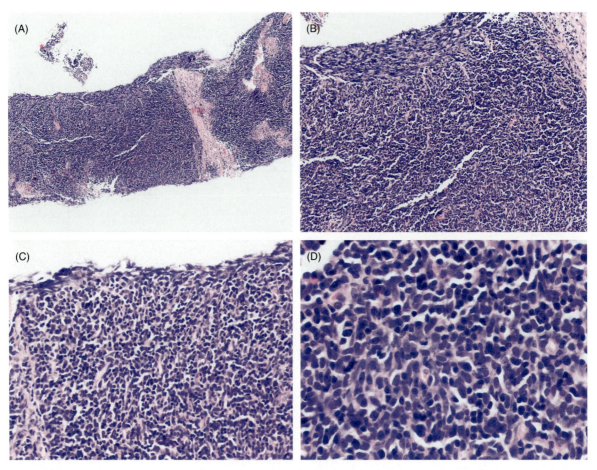

Illustrative case 3 (A–E) H&E sections from this core biopsy show a diffuse infiltrate apparently composed of small to medium-sized lymphocytes. There is prominent traction artefact (B,C). High power examination (D,E) reveals a population of slightly larger cells with pale nuclei and multiple small nucleoli. Immunohistochemistry shows CD3-positive T cells (F) which express TdT (G) and show a high proliferation fraction with MIB1 (H). Cytokeratin staining with CK19 (I) and AE1/AE3 (J) reveal that the larger pale cells are epithelial in nature and form a network running throughout the biopsy. The epithelial cells in this network also express CD20 (K).

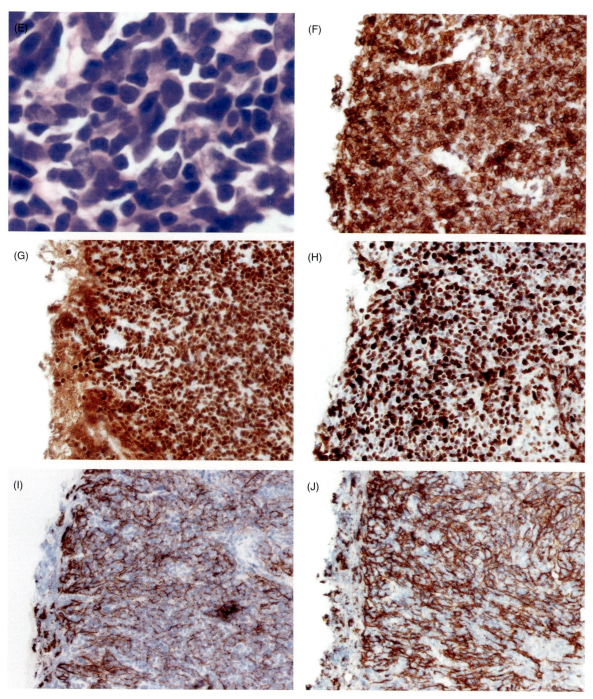

Illustrative case 3 (cont.)

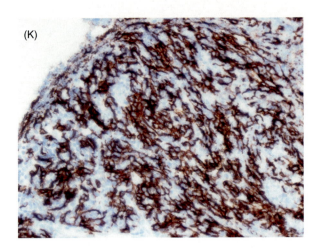

(K)

Illustrative case 3 (cont.)

Index

8p11 myeloproliferative syndrome, 116
acid-fast bacilli, 12
adenocarcinoma, 94, 144
adult T cell leukemia/lymphoma
    (ATLL), 120, 126
ALK-positive large B cell lymphoma,
    87, 90, 129
amyloid, 134
anaplastic large cell lymphoma (ALCL),
    19, 39, 93, 120, 149, 152
    ALK negative, 120, 125, 129
    ALK positive, 93, 120, 124, 128
    Hodgkin-like, 129
    lymphohistiocytic variant, 129
    small cell variant, 129
angioimmunoblastic T cell lymphoma
    (AITL), 120, 121, 129
    perifollicular pattern in, 129
apoptosis, 17, 18, 38, 66, 74, 92
asteroid bodies, 12

B cell lymphoma unclassifiable
    with features intermediate
    between DLBCL and BL, 71,
    74, 92
B cell lymphoma unclassifiable with
    features intermediate between
    DLBCL and CHL, 39, 92
bcl-2 translocation, 52, 71, 74, 90, 91
bcl-6 rearrangement, 71, 74
Burkitt lymphoma (BL), 66, 71–74,
    92, 112

carcinoma, 92, 136, 144, 149
    CD138 positivity in, 137
caseous necrosis, 12
Castleman disease, 13–17, 25
    hyaline-vascular subtype, 13–14
    plasma cell subtype, 15–17
CCND1 translocation, 67, 92, 94, 134
CD117, 93, 134
CD1a, 4, 21, 123, 144
CD30, 20, 39
    in CHL, 37
    in germ cell tumors, 93
    in NLPHL, 47
    in normal paracortex, 5
CD57, 43, 47
centroblasts, 1, 45, 52, 56, 88, 148
centrocytes, 1, 45, 52, 79, 105

chronic lymphocytic leukemia/
    small lymphocytic lymphoma
    (CLL/SLL), 54, 66, 79, 105–108
    CD5 negative, 107
    Richter's transformation of, 108
classical Hodgkin lymphoma (CHL), 19,
    27, 35–39, 43, 91, 126, 128, 129, 152
    interfollicular, 36, 39
c-myc translocation, 71, 91, 92
CXCL13, 1, 120, 122, 127, 128
cyclin D1, 1, 52, 79, 81, 92, 94, 105, 112,
    134, 137
cytokeratins, 93, 114, 149
    in metastatic carcinoma, 144
    in plasma cell neoplasms, 134, 137
cytotoxic markers, 18, 20, 47, 93, 124,
    126, 149

dermatopathic lymphadenopathy,
    20–1, 39, 123
desmoplakin, 144
diffuse large B cell lymphoma
    (DLBCL), 19, 39, 56, 71, 87–94,
    129, 134, 148
    CD20 negative, 94
    CD5 positive, 94
    cyclin D1 positive, 94
    interfollicular, 93
double hit lymphoma, 91

EBER, 20, 28, 37, 38, 43, 66, 67, 71, 74,
    75, 90, 92, 93, 122, 124, 125, 126,
    127, 128, 136, 137
EBV-positive DLBCL of the elderly, 87
EBV-LMP1, 39
enteropathy-associated T cell
    lymphoma (EATL), 120
epithelioid histiocytes, 12, 65, 120, 122,
    123, 128, 129
Epstein–Barr virus (EBV), 19
extramedullary plasmacytoma, 134
extranodal marginal zone lymphoma,
    see MALT lymphoma
extranodal NK/T cell lymphoma, nasal
    type, 120

fascin, 144
FGFR1 abnormality, 116
follicular colonization, 82
follicular dendritic cell sarcoma, 144

follicular dendritic cells (FDCs), 1, 5,
    14, 17, 43, 47, 66, 112, 121, 122
follicular helper T cells (T_{FH}), 1, 120,
    121, 122
follicular lymphoma (FL), 43, 52–56,
    66, 79, 105, 112
    bcl-2 negative, 56
    floral pattern, 56
    grade 56
    interfollicular component, 56
    inverted pattern, 56
    signet ring, 56
    with marginal zone differentiation, 56
    with monocytoid differentiation, 56
follicular lysis, 5

germ cell tumor, 93, 144, 148
germinal centers, 1, 5, 12, 52
    in Castleman disease, 14, 15
    in marginal zone lymphoma, 79
    streaming of, 5, 55
granulomas, 12, 13, 26, 36, 43
    in DLBCL, 94
    in peripheral T cell lymphomas, 123

hematopathologist, 7
hallmark cells, 124, 125
Hassall's corpuscles, 114
HHV8, 14, 15, 28, 136, 146, 148
histiocytic sarcoma, 93, 144
HIV (human immunodeficiency virus),
    15, 17, 29, 134, 137, 138
Hodgkin cells, 19, 35, 36, 39, 91

ICOS, 1, 120, 127, 128
infectious mononucleosis (IM), 19–20,
    39, 93, 125
interdigitating dendritic cell
    sarcoma, 144
interdigitating dendritic cells (IDCs), 3,
    21, 123
intravascular large B cell lymphoma, 87

Kaposi sarcoma (KS), 17, 148
Kaposi sarcoma virus (KSHV, HHV8),
    15, 17, 25
Kikuchi lymphadenitis (KL), 17–19, 120

Langerhans cell histiocytosis, 144
Langerhans cells, 3, 6, 144, 145

langerin (CD207), 144
Langhans giant cells, 12
LP cells, 43, 45, 47, 105
lymphoblastic leukemia/lymphoma
    (LBL), 74, 105, 112–116
  B cell, 66, 112
  T cell, 112, 114, 116, 152
lymphoblasts, 66, 112
lymphoepithelial lesions, 52, 56, 79
lymphoplasmacytic lymphoma (LPL),
    66, 79–82, 105, 134

MALT lymphoma, 52, 56, 79
mantle cell lymphoma (MCL), 1, 52,
    64–67, 74, 79, 94, 105
  blastoid variant, 66, 112
  CD5 negative, 67
  cyclin D1 negative, 67
  pleomorphic variant, 66, 92
mantle zone, 1, 52, 56
  "onion-skin" pattern, 14, 16
marginal zone lymphoma (MZL), 66,
    79–82, 105, 121
  with plasma cell differentiation,
    134
melanoma, 93, 136, 144, 149, 152
  amelanotic, 147
  CD138 positivity in, 137
Merkel cell carcinoma, 129
monocytoid B cells, 12, 23, 28
MYD88 L265P mutation, 81
myeloid sarcoma, 93, 112, 144
  monocytic differentiation in, 144
  plasmacytoid dendritic cell
    differentiation in, 144
myeloperoxidase (MPO), 18, 29, 115

nodular lymphocyte predominant
    Hodgkin lymphoma (NLPHL), 39,
    43–47, 52, 105

OCT–3/4, 93, 148

paracortex, 1, 5
  in dermatopathic lymphadenopathy,
    21
  in infectious mononucleosis, 19, 20
paraimmunoblasts, 54, 66, 105, 108
PCR
  in DLBCL, 94
  in follicular lymphoma, 52, 56
  in infectious mononucleosis, 20
  in plasma cell neoplasms, 134, 137
PD1, 1, 43, 47, 120, 122, 127, 128, 129
peripheral T cell lymphoma not
    otherwise specified (PTCL-NOS),
    93, 120
  CD30 negative, 120
  CD30 positive, 120
  follicular variant, 56, 129
peripheral T cell lymphomas, 120–129
PLAP, 93, 146, 148
plasma cell myeloma, 134
plasma cell neoplasms (PCNs), 79,
    134–137
plasmablastic lymphoma, 87, 134, 136,
    149, 152
plasmablasts
  in plasma cell Castleman disease, 17
plasmacytoid dendritic cells (PDC), 14,
    17, 18, 28, 29
primary effusion lymphoma (PEL),
    136, 152

primary follicles, 5
primary mediastinal large
    B cell lymphoma (PMLBCL),
    87, 90
progressive transformation
    of germinal centers
    (PTGC), 47
proliferation centers, 79, 105
prolymphocytes, 105

Reed–Sternberg cells, 35, 36, 37,
    43, 128
  in ALCL, 124
  in ATLL, 126
  in T cell lymphoma, 120
  in viral infections, 125

sarcoid, 12, 23
sarcoma, 144, 148
Schaumann bodies, 12
seminoma, 148, 152
small cell carcinoma of the lung, 129,
    144
SOX11, 65, 66, 67, 74, 92, 105

T cell/histiocyte-rich large B cell
    lymphoma (THRLBCL), 46, 47,
    87, 129
tadpole sign, 14
TdT, 66, 67, 74, 105, 112, 114, 115, 127,
    128, 129, 130
tennis racquet sign, 14
toxoplasmosis, 12–13
tuberculosis, 12, 23

Ziehl–Neelsen staining, 12